Intrapartum Care

Edited by
Kathleen Kendall-Tackett, PhD, IBCLC, FAPA
& Scott Sherwood, BS

All royalties go to the
U.S. Lactation Consultant Association.

Praeclarus Press, LLC

Praeclarus Press, LLC
2504 Sweetgum Lane
Amarillo, Texas 79124 USA
806-367-9950
www.PraeclarusPress.com

DISCLAIMER

The information contained in this publication is advisory only and is not intended to replace sound clinical judgment or individualized patient care. The author disclaims all warranties, whether expressed or implied, including any warranty as the quality, accuracy, safety, or suitability of this information for any particular purpose.

ISBN 978-1-939807-36-6

Cover Design: Ken Tackett

Acquisition & Development: Kathleen Kendall-Tackett & Scott Sherwood

Copy Editing: Chris Tackett

Layout & Design: Nelly Murariu

Operations: Scott Sherwood

Contents

What Happens to Breastfeeding When Mothers Lie Back?

Clinical Applications of Biological Nurturing

Suzanne Colson, RGN, RM, PhD[1]

Keywords: Biological Nurturing, primitive neonatal reflexes, mother's posture

Human neonates are born with an innate ability to find the breast, latch, and feed. Unfortunately, some of these very reflexes can also hinder babies' efforts to breastfeed, depending on the mother's posture. This article provides a brief overview on the mechanisms of Biological Nurturing™ (BN) and describes how practitioners can help mothers trigger innate feeding mechanisms so that they do not become barriers to breastfeeding.

From a survival standpoint, it makes evolutionary sense that neonates be born with a number of simple, innate movements enabling them to find the food source, latch on, and feed. With the 20th century rise of bottle-feeding,

1 Akinsanya Scholar 2007, honorary senior lecturer at Canterbury Christ Church University and a co–founder of The Nurturing Project

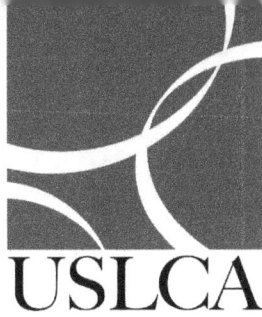

however, we lost that sense of the babies' ability to find the breast. More concerning are subtle ways bottle-feeding norms still influence advice breastfeeding mothers receive. The current mainstream approach is that mothers need to sit upright to latch their babies (UNICEF UK et al., 2008). Inherent in this approach is that mothers must counteract gravity by applying pressure along the baby's back.

Indeed, our findings suggest that when mothers sit upright, or even when they lie on their sides, gravity pulls the baby away from the mother's body. To counteract gravitational forces, mothers hold their babies close; these holds often suppress, limit, or even waste innate baby-feeding reflexes. In fact, these same reflexes may actually become barriers (rather than aides) to latch and sustain milk transfer (Colson et al., 2008).

The Role of the Primitive Neonatal Reflexes

Our research revealed that during breastfeeding, babies use 20 primitive neonatal reflexes (PNRs). PNRs are indicators of neurological function, and are an important component of biological nurturing (BN). Surprisingly, many of the 20 PNRs described during the work appeared to have a dual role—either helping or hindering breastfeeding.

An unexpected finding from this study was that the mother's posture influenced the role that the PNRs played. As soon as the mothers lie back, they look comfortable, relaxed, and focused upon their babies—often smiling, giggling, and oblivious to the world. The baby finds the breast using his inborn reflexes that now look smooth and purposeful. Because the strength of reaction is somewhat blunted by gravity, the baby reflexes appear to aid neonatal locomotion, leading to latching behaviors, self-attachment, and good milk transfer. (Colson et al., 2008). It is as if the position the mother sits in could transform breastfeeding from a method reliant upon skills into a relationship.

In BN, mothers neither sit upright nor do they lie on their sides or backs. Instead, at the start of a feed, they lean back in semi-reclined postures, usually placing the baby on top of their bodies, so the entire frontal aspect of the baby's body is facing, touching, and closely applied to their body curves or to a part of the environment (Colson, 2005a, 2005b; Colson et al., 2008). The movement is in the pelvis and an understanding of pelvic anatomy underpins using BN. We formulated scientific definitions for the mother's feeding position based upon bony pelvic reliance and amount of back support.

The Role of the Bony Pelvis

Kapandji (1974), a French orthopedic surgeon, integrated and illustrated complex physiology and mechanical functioning of joints and muscles within the anatomical context. His explanations and illustrations, together with those from recent English midwifery textbooks, provide the basis for understanding the difference between upright and laid–back sitting postures.

Pelvic Sitting Support

When sitting upright or leaning slightly forward, the body mass is supported evenly by the two ischial tuberosities. In ischial sitting postures, for example, those used to drive a car, ride a bike, or to work at the computer, the weight of the trunk sits firmly upon a solid base, either a chair, or a seat (Kapandji, 1974). Bodyweight is placed equally on both ischial tuberosities; the thighs are parallel to the floor and ideally, the seat height permits the feet to rest flat on the floor. The body leans forward from the hips when necessary but does not curve at shoulders or neck. Kapandji (1974, p. 112) calls this the "typist position," characterizing it as fraught with potential for muscular fatigue and the most difficult body posture to sustain.

In contrast, when sitting laid-back, for example, sprawled on a chair or sofa while watching television, the back of the chair or sofa always supports the trunk. Bony pelvic reliance comprises the posterior surface of the sacrum and the coccyx with limited ischial support. Kapandji (1974, p. 112) terms this posture the "position of relaxation." It is an in-between posture neither sitting bolt upright nor flat-lying. Kapandjii states that this position can be achieved with the help of cushions or specially designed chairs, but our results show that mothers do not need any equipment to sit in this position. Figure 1 summarizes these differences comparing an adaptation of Kapandji's "typist's position" with his "position of relaxation."

Figure 2 illustrates these postures in live mothers. The bottle-feeding mother on the left is ischial sitting, upright at 90°, as is the breastfeeding mother in the middle. On the right, the same breastfeeding mother has changed to sacral sitting and is semi-reclined at a 35° angle.

Maternal comfort mechanisms

All mothers experience a wide range of challenges to their personal comfort right after birth. The abrupt change in body shape can be a real shock and sometimes body parts feel sensitive, ache, or are sore. This can be compounded by abdominal pain if the mother has had a caesarean birth, or perineal pain if she has had an episiotomy or assisted delivery. A mother may also have pain from sore nipples or engorgement, and some also complain of neck tension and shoulder pain. This may be because it is difficult to maintain the upright position for long periods of time (Kapandji, 1974).

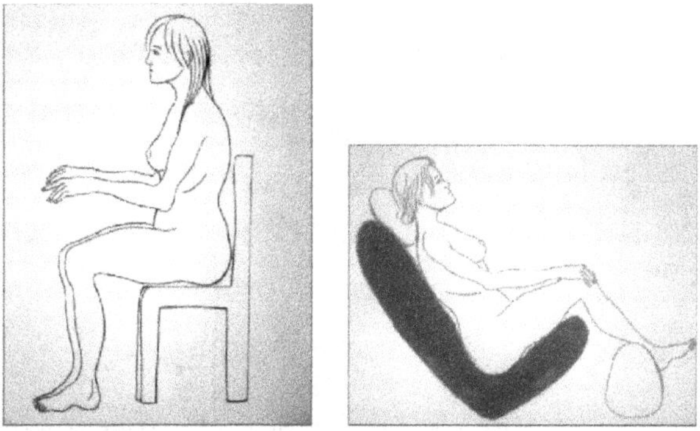

Figure 1. Contrast the typist's position (ischial sitting) with the position of relaxation (sacral sitting).

Laid–back breastfeeding, by definition, means that every part of the mother's body—importantly, her head, neck, shoulders, upper and lower back are relaxed. Mothers often say that as soon as they sit back, the shoulder and neck tension melt away. Nipple pain is often alleviated immediately, and this may happen because gravity is not dragging the baby down the upright maternal midriff. Mothers also have increased freedom of movement as one or both hands are free; their bodies hold the baby not their arms. Figure 3 compares maternal body support in upright postures with BN postures

Does this mean that mothers should never initiate breastfeeding in upright postures? From a practical standpoint, no. Human mothers and babies are extremely versatile, able to breastfeed in many different positions, and it would not be helpful to prescribe laid-back postures as the only way to initiate breastfeeding. Millions of mothers have obviously been able to breastfeed while sitting up. But there are some limitations to that approach. In our study, observations for the first episode demonstrated that 12 of the 27 breastfeeding mothers who sat upright latched their baby successfully onto the breast with good milk transfer. However, only a quarter of them (N=3) were pain–free; the other nine mothers modified their baby's positions, their own postures, or both in subsequent episodes to achieve an increase in comfort.

In contrast, the laid–back BN posture immediately changed things. It opened the mother's body which gave the baby more space to maneuver. Importantly, mothers'

Figure 2. Contrast mothers sitting bolt upright (left and center photos) with the mother sitting semi–reclined (right photo).

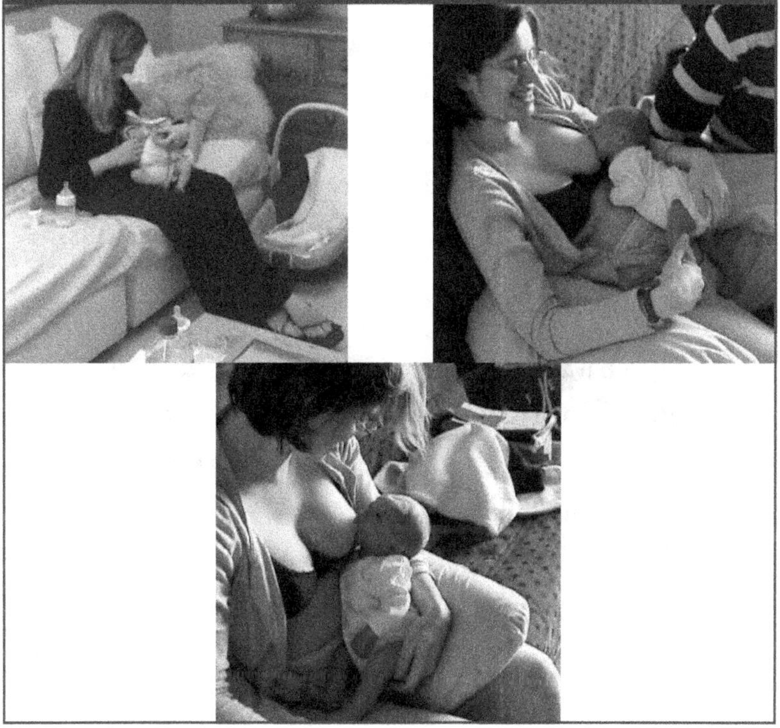

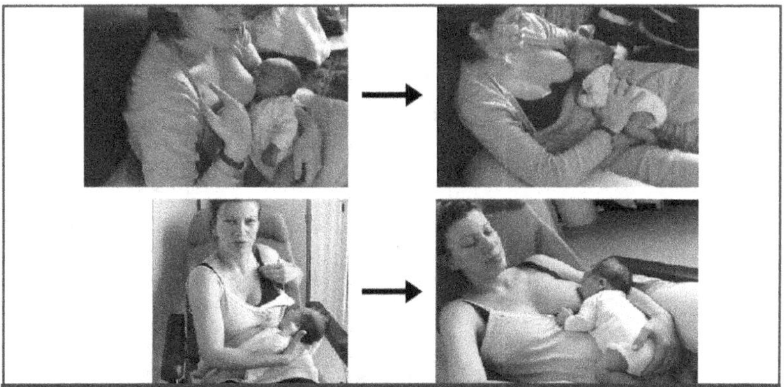

Figure 3. Maternal body support from upright to BN postures

bodies were fully supported and they often had both hands free because they no longer needed to hold the baby applying pressure along the baby's back, head, or neck; gravity helped keep the baby on the mother's body. In addition, when mothers initiate breastfeeding while sitting upright, they may be faced with more direct instruction and intervention than when they are left alone to quietly discover each other, as this mother describes.

> *Dear Suzanne,*
>
> *My son was placed to my breast shortly after the birth and fed for about 35 minutes, and it was fabulous. The midwife was very relaxed and simply placed him there and let him do his own thing, while I laid back and relaxed! I decided there and then that breastfeeding was definitely for me, but was very apprehensive as I had heard so many negative things regarding it, and I did not know anyone who had been successful for any length of time. I am certain that if my midwife had not been so natural and chilled out about this first feed, things would have been very different. I was moved to the postnatal ward a few hours after the birth. It was horrendous. Nurses standing guard and scrutinizing every move I made breast-wise! It was here that I heard the mantra "tummy to mummy, nipple to nose" spoken aloud. I had read about it before the birth, but didn't realize it was almost treated as the law! I hate those words now; I found myself repeating them in my head, and didn't dare deviate. I was also told to sit bolt upright ... I was intimidated to say the least when a line up of 3 nurses stood in front of me watching me trying*

> *to force my baby to latch on. They said I couldn't go home until I could manage to feed him ok, but I so wanted to be out of there. I tried to let him find his way to the nipple and was immediately berated for it! Now you can see why I would have appreciated simply being told that there are alternative ways to breastfeed! The hospital staff was obsessed with breastfeeding without seeming to offer any practical advice except for the instructions printed in the government leaflets. I have learned now that, as a mother, your instincts CAN be trusted, and that your baby is well equipped to feed himself given half a chance. I just needed someone to tell me this at the time! Thanks again [for explaining BN which] has given me so much reassurance and a lot more confidence about things. I hope I can pass this on to any new mums I come into contact with through my peer supporting role in the future.*

Is BN Species–Specific?: Directions for Future Research

This initial research on the mechanisms of BN raises some interesting questions, such as could BN postures and positions be species specific? Human infants develop as quadrupeds; locomotion is first achieved through crawling. The human baby struggles to a semi-upright sitting posture from 4 to 7 months of age, beginning to toddle erect when they are about a year old. Taken together these facts suggest a strong developmental argument: our babies, like some of our quadruped mammalian cousins, would biologically commence life as abdominal, or what I call frontal feeders. The human upright struggle against gravity is progressive suggesting that phylogenetically, our babies would be semi–upright to feed, supported by a gentle maternal body slope. If being human involves retracing our phylogenetic history, as Peiper (1963) suggests, then during the first year of life, BN laid–back maternal postures enabling full neonatal frontal feeding positions may be a species–specific positional choice, aiding breastfeeding initiation.

Conclusions

The results of our research have had an amazing impact upon my practice. If you are interested in applying BN in your practice, here are some guidelines that will help you do so.

Clinical Applications I: Using BN to support a mother getting started with breastfeeding.

You may want to:

1. Explain that for her, a BN posture is one where her back touches and is supported by the back of the chair or sofa; her own comfort is the priority. Tell her there is not one "correct" breastfeeding position and she might like to try feeding her baby in the same positions she uses to watch television.
2. Explain that her body supports the baby, not her arms or pillows. However, pillows can sometimes help to support her own arms, upper back, head and or shoulders.
3. Share that mothers often sacrifice their own personal comfort for a good latch. This may increase fatigue and should be avoided. Tell her that an important part of your role is to check that every part of her body is supported.
4. Help her place the baby on top of her body in a position where every aspect of the baby's body can brush up against one of her body curves or a part of the environment, such as a blanket, bed clothes, or the bed or chair. This is particularly important for the baby's thighs, feet tops and soles.
5. Share that a baby often uses inborn reflexes to move into a position similar to the way he was lying in the womb. This point of continuity may be comforting to both mother and baby.

Clinical Applications II: Problems such as latch refusal, sore nipples & breast fullness.

You may want to:

1. Suggest that she does BN when the baby is in sleep states. This entails picking up the sleeping baby without waking him and laying him on top of mother's body in BN postures/position. We have not looked at the effects of behavioral state in this paper. However, it is well known that reflex actions can be released in sleep states and an entire chapter is devoted to this important subject in Colson (2010).

2. Use BN as a test for tongue tie before you separate baby and mother to make a physical assessment of the baby's mouth. Gravity always brings the tongue and chin forward during BN.

General Observations. Be aware that BN:

1. Is not a maternal flat-lying posture and the reasons for this are discussed in detail in Colson (2010).

2. Is usually carried out when mothers and babies are lightly dressed except for the first hours following birth.

3. Maternal postures open up a wide variety of baby positions. Like the hands of a clock, the baby can approach the breast from any angle. This means that the baby does not always lead in with the chin. Rather the entire trigeminal facial area may bob against the mother's breast. Attachment is not always asymmetrical.

4. Baby positions promote self attachment but not always. Sometimes the mother needs to help. During self-attachment, the baby's body is not always in a straight line.

5. Attachment can initially look like nipple sucking and as long as there is good milk transfer and there is no pain, this more superficial BN attachment works well.

References

Colson, S. (2005a). Maternal breastfeeding positions, have we got it right? (1). *The Practising Midwife, 8,* 10, 24–27.

Colson, S. (2005b). Maternal breastfeeding positions, have we got it right? (2). *The Practising Midwife, 8,* 11, 29–32.

Colson, S. (2010). *An introduction to biological nurturing: New angles on breastfeeding.* Amarillo, TX: Hale Publishing.

Colson, S.D., Meek J.H., & Hawdon, J.M. (2008). Optimal positions for the release of primitive neonatal reflexes stimulating breastfeeding. *Early Human Development, 84,* 441–449. Available online at http://linkinghub.elsevier.com/retrieve/pii/S0378378207002423

Kapandji, I.A. (1974). *The physiology of the joints. Vol.3. The trunk and the vertebral column (2nd ed.).*Edinburgh: Churchill Livingstone.

Peiper, A. (1963). *Cerebral function in infancy and childhood (3rd ed.)* In B. Nagler & H. Nagler (Trans.). New York: Consultants Bureau.

UNICEF UK Baby Friendly Initiative & the Health Promotion Agency for Northern Ireland. (2008). *Teaching breastfeeding skills* [videocassette]. The Health Promotion Agency for Northern Ireland 18 Omeau Avenue Belfast BT2 8HS cover available on line at http://www.healthpromotionagency.org.uk/Resources/breastfeeding/pdfs/Breastfeeding_DVD_Case.pdf

USLCA

Facilitating Autonomous Infant Hand Use During Breastfeeding

Catherine Watson Genna, BS, IBCLC, RLC[1]
Diklah Barak, BOT[2]

Keywords: breastfeeding, laid-back breastfeeding, infant hand, infant feeding behaviors

Infant ability to find and attach to the breast has only been recently appreciated. When mothers are in reclined, laid-back, or Biological Nurturing™ positions, the mothers' bodies provide optimal support for their infants, which releases infant instinctive feeding behaviors. One type of instinctive behavior that infants reveal is their deliberate use of their hands to locate, move, and shape the nipple area. In this article, we provide photographic evidence of several infant hand-use strategies, as well as information on how professionals and mothers can elicit, support, and modify these behaviors when needed. The videos that are referenced in this article can be found here: https://www.youtube.com/playlist?list=PLNQYGRLLfeFTBiiC61K-L98iTm1W6nkFq

Mothers are often taught to hold their babies' hands when latching them on to avoid them "getting in the

1 Private practice, New York City
2 Private practice, New York City

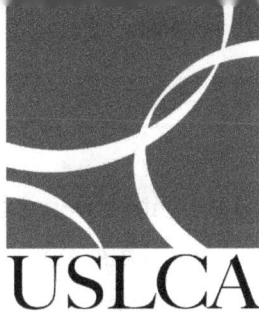

way." Historically, infant movements were thought to be random and purposeless. This may be because infants are often studied in solitary conditions, separated from their mothers. Infants studied at their mother's breast produce predictable movements (Prechtl, 1958), but it is difficult to prove that infants' movements are intentional. Lew and Butterworth (1995, p. 456) found that infants fed sugar solution bring their hands to the breast, but in the absence of the breast, this posture is likely to result in hand-mouth contacts.

When researchers photographed and videotaped infants, they were able to analyze movements that occur closely in time. Butterworth and Hopkins (1988) stated that infant hand-to-mouth movements seem to be deliberate but not well coordinated.

> *The hand-mouth coordination has all the characteristics of a goal-directed act, which only occasionally fulfils its intended outcome because it is unskilled. The fact that the mouth opens before the arm moves suggests that the mouth actually anticipates the arrival of the hand rather than simply acting as the passive terminus for the movement (p. 311).*

Butterworth hypothesized that infants used hand-to-mouth movements to regulate their state and to self-calm (p. 313), but not as part of the sucking reflex, as he saw little finger sucking in his films of newborns.

These behaviors also appear in utero. Researchers used ultrasound to study the development of motor skills in fetuses of various gestational ages. Miller et al. (2003) noted that the fetus almost invariably touched the face or mouth before swallowing amniotic fluid. Sparling et al. (1999) noted that movements of 21 low-risk (healthy) fetuses appeared non-random, and changed from month-to-month. Duration of hand-to-mouth movements were greatest at 20 weeks gestation, and then increased again after birth. This decrease, then reappearance is "consistent with developmental curves where a movement disappears to reappear in a more advanced pattern"(p. 35).

Van der Meer et al. (1995) demonstrated that infants use vision to guide antigravity hand movements. The infant subjects lifted their weighted hands only when they could see them, either directly or on a video monitor. Bringing infants to the breast with their hands hugging the breast keeps the hands in the peripheral vision. Figure 1a shows an infant in this position, looking intently at the

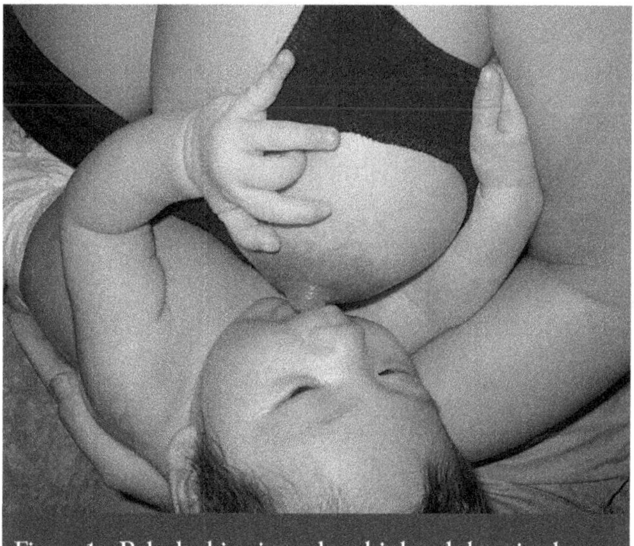

Figure 1a. Baby looking intently at his hands hugging breast.

breast before attaching (1b). Having the hands in this position also helps stabilize the neck and shoulder girdle by adducting (pulling together) the shoulder blades. Hand movements are also stronger when the arms are raised rather than held at the infant's sides (Prechtl, 1958).

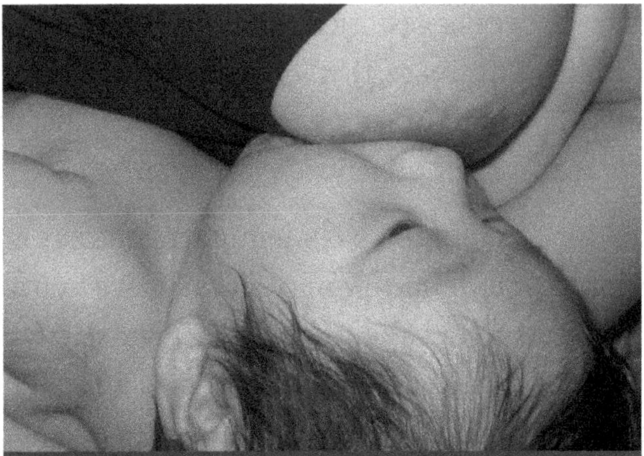

Figure 1b. Latching with tongue down.

Mother-infant skin-to-skin contact influenced maternal oxytocin levels in another study (Mathieson et al., 2001). Newborns in this study invariably oriented to the breast and used massage-like hand movements on the mother's breast and nipple area, which both caused increased maternal oxytocin levels, and caused the nipple areolar area to become erect and more prominent to facilitate latch. Ransjo-Arvedson et al. (2001) found differences in newborn feeding behaviors in those exposed to labor analgesia, including IV pethidine (meperidine) and/or epidural bupivacaine. Only 40% of drug-exposed infants attached to the breast, and all of those who latched massaged their mother's breast significantly longer than infants born to unmedicated mothers.

A classic study demonstrated that touch to different parts of the infant's face stimulated specific movement patterns (Prechtl, 1958). When infants were touched on the corner of their mouth and cheek, they started side-to-side scanning or rooting movements, which Prechtl called the pendulous orientating response. The newborns rubbed their faces on the stimulus from one corner of their mouth to the other corner of their mouth. Infants use scanning to search the mother's chest for her breast. This particular response was interesting because it was the only one Prechtl identified that did not accommodate over repetition. Other reflex responses become inhibited in the brain over repeated stimuli, whereas alternating repetitive stimuli to the corners of the mouth provoked repeated side-to-side head movement. This behavior continued until the perioral area came into contact with the nipple, when the baby would gape, search with the tongue for the nipple, and pull the nipple into the mouth. The researchers most efficiently stimulated gape (mouth opening) at the philtrum, the area between the upper lip and nose. In contrast, when only the lower lip was stimulated, babies flexed their heads and moved their lower lips downward.

Mathieson et al. (2001) found that newborns used their hands, as well as their lips and tongue, to draw the nipple into their mouths, a response which persists in infants until about 3-4 months of age, and can be used to help infants learn to breastfeed (Smillie, 2008). Paul, Papousek, and colleagues (1996) studied feeding behaviors of infants monthly from 2 weeks to 26 weeks, and found that pre-feeding motor movements decreased between 18 and 26 weeks of age. After studying 20 infants over 6 months, they concluded that infants demonstrated a "finely organized behavioral pattern" (Paul et al., 1996, p. 572).

The position the mother is in can obstruct or facilitate infant movements. Colson et al. (2008) demonstrated that infant and maternal feeding-related reflexes were facilitated by the mother being in a semi-reclined position, allowing the baby to be on its abdomen. Anti-gravity movements, such as scanning and head righting, were identified as particularly important in finding and attaching to the breast. Maternal semi-reclining positions are also more ergonomic for the mother, freeing her arms from the need to hold the baby's weight to her body against the pull of gravity. Further information on this technique can be found at http://biologicalnurturing.com.

We've observed that semi-reclining improves access to the nipple as the breast lifts off the postpartum belly. In the laid-back position, gravity supports the baby's weight on the mother's abdomen or chest, providing the vital stability that allows for better motoric function. This allows the infants muscles to work in feeding rather than attempting to stabilize their body position. Furthermore, if the infant attempts to latch when his body is sidelying and misses, gravity pulls him away from the breast, whereas if the infant misses the breast while prone, gravity pulls him toward the breast.

How Infants Use their Hands at the Breast

It is well recognized that infants put their hands to the breast. But it is less well-known whether their hand movements are intentional. Almost all breastfeeding instructions include restraining the baby's arms. However, we've observed that if left unhindered, infants from birth to at least 3-4 months of age use their hands during the attachment process. How the infant uses the hands and arms depends partly on the orientation of the infant's face to the breast. If the face is touching the breast, infants may use their hands to push or pull the breast to make the nipple accessible to the mouth, or to shape a better-defined teat. If the face is not touching the breast, infants may use their arms to push away, perhaps to get a look at the nipple location, or may search with the hands for the nipple and close on it or just below it. Once the hand finds the nipple, the baby mouths the hand, calms, and then often moves the hand away and latches on to the same spot.

The following examples have been captured in photographs and videos. Figure 2a shows the infant resisting the mother's attempt to push the breast toward his mouth. Once he is attached, he relaxes his hand (Figure 2b). The infant in Figure 3 (a and b) is tongue-tied and cannot extend the tongue enough to grasp the breast well, so she uses her hands to pull the breast into her mouth. On video clip a, a one-month-old baby who has been latching shallowly (to only the nipple) with "traditional" latch techniques, is given more autonomy at the breast. She brings her hand to the areola, sucks her hand, comes away from the breast for perhaps a better look or to re-adjust her position, then comes back to the breast. The author (CWG) helps the mother bring the baby closer to help her attach more deeply. In video b, the same baby moves the hand away and latches, when brought close enough so that she feels the breast with her face. In Figure 4a and 4b (video c), a 14-day-old infant shapes the breast with his hand, using the technique illustrated in Rebecca Glover's video, *Follow me Mum!*

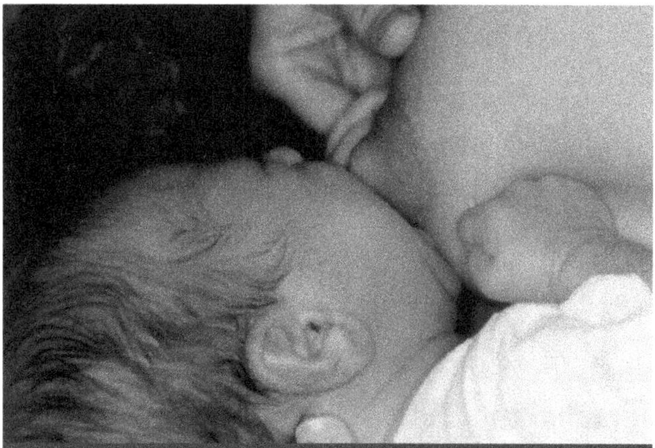

Figure 2a. Baby resists maternal breast pushing.

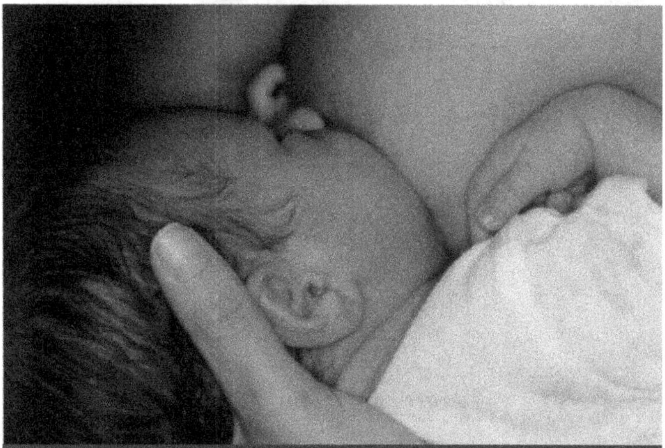

Figure 2b. He relaxes his hand once latched.

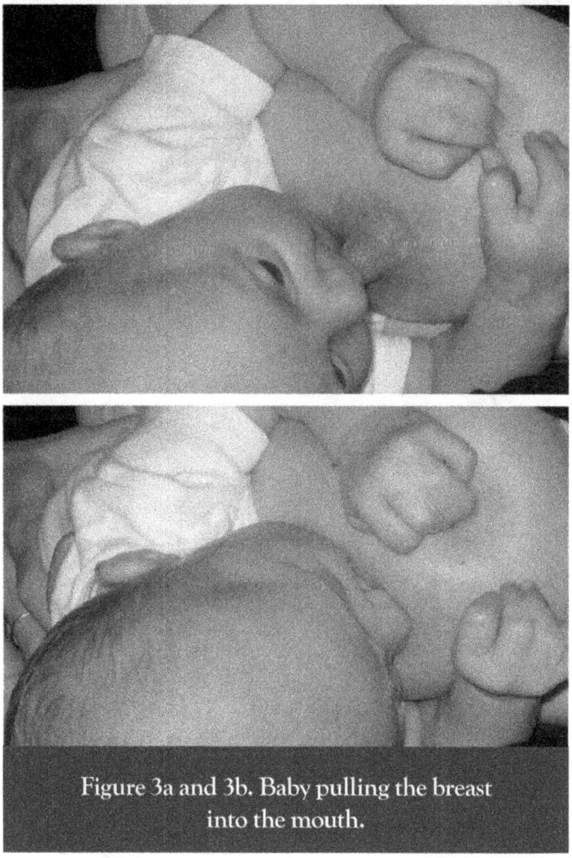

Figure 3a and 3b. Baby pulling the breast into the mouth.

Video Captions

In video 2a, the baby pushes off the breast and immediately returns to the spot her hand rested on before, and on video 2b, teaching the mom to use cheek to breast to help her baby relax her hands and use oral searching (see Figure 7). In video 4a and 4b, the baby spontaneously and repeatedly shapes the breast to make the areola bulge out until he can orally grasp the breast (see Figure 4).

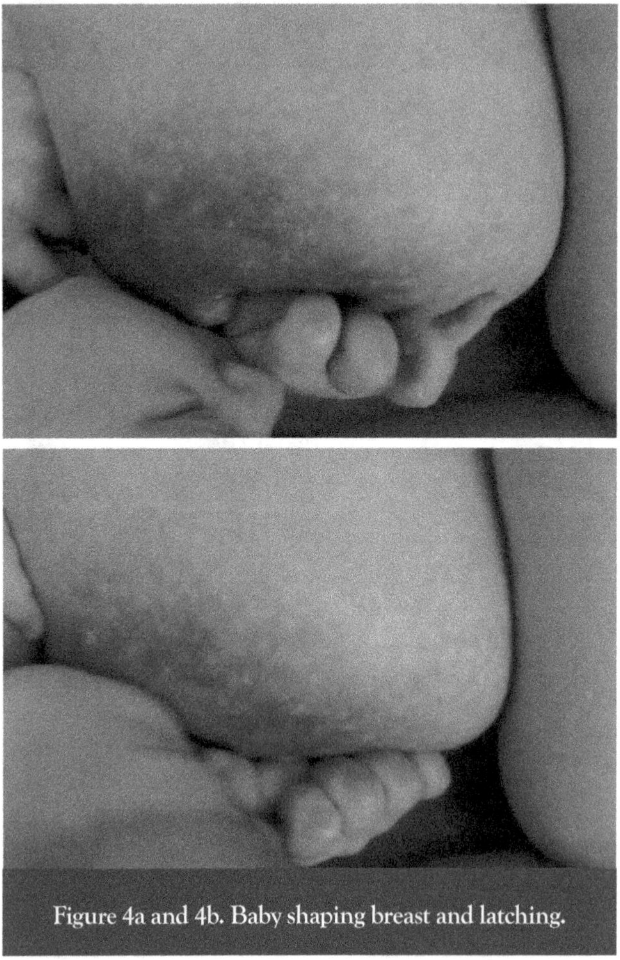

Figure 4a and 4b. Baby shaping breast and latching.

How to Facilitate Skillful Infant Hand Use

Start with a semi-reclined, comfortable maternal position with the infant snuggled close to the mom so that the baby's body is completely supported, as in Figure 5.

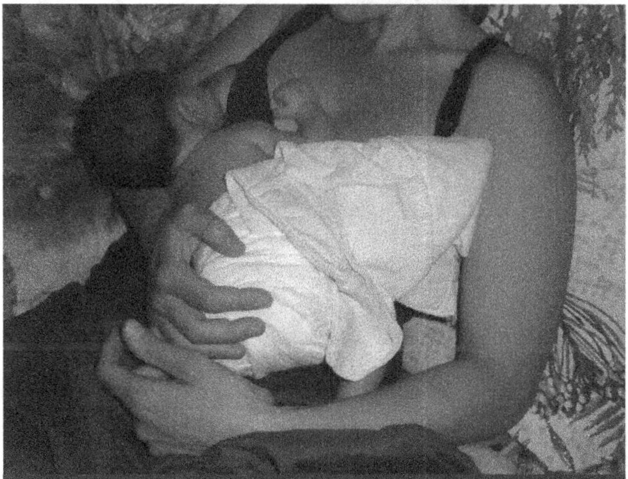

Figure 5. Laid-back breastfeeding position

Bringing the infant's arms around to "hug" the breast allows them to stay in the line of sight, which improves motor strength and precision. Avoid restricting the baby's use of their hands by swaddling, holding the arms, or trapping them in the mother's cleavage. If a laid-back breastfeeding position is not possible, using a cradle hold, and snuggling the baby's belly very close to the mom's body helps the infant access and use his hands.

Many infants respond with mouth gape, tongue protrusion, and latch when placed with their chin or face to the breast. Placing the baby's body so the chin is snuggled in to the areola, and the philtrum touches the nipple elicits the widest gape response, consistent with Prechtl's findings (1958). Figures 6 a and b illustrate the infant response to this appropriate stimulus.

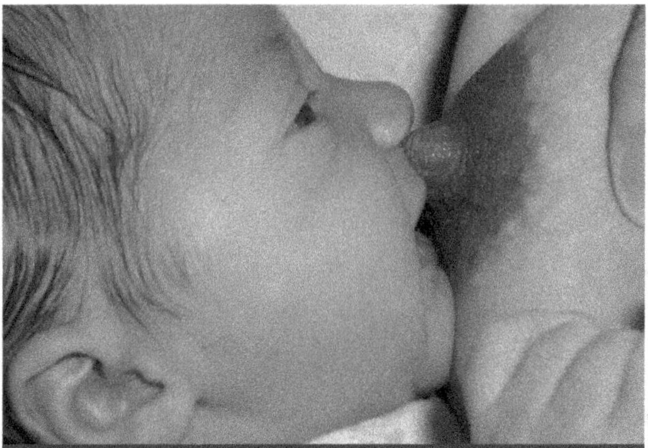

Figure 6a. Chin to breast and nipple to philtrum

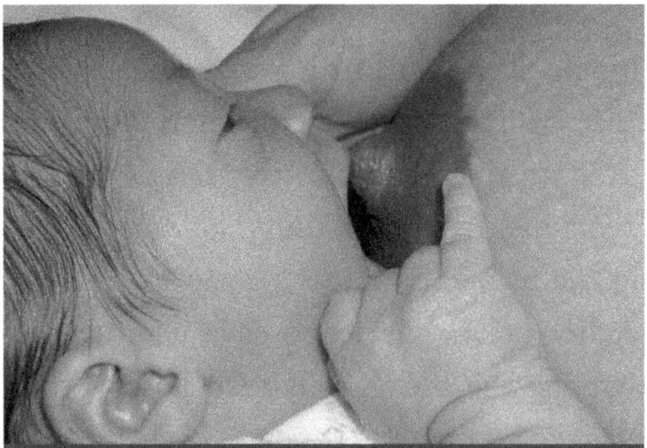

Figure 6b. Resultant large gape

Some infants respond better to positioning with their cheek on the breast just above the areola so they can root or scan down to the nipple, as in Figure 7.

Other infants need to begin their behavioral feeding sequence from "start" and find the breast independently.

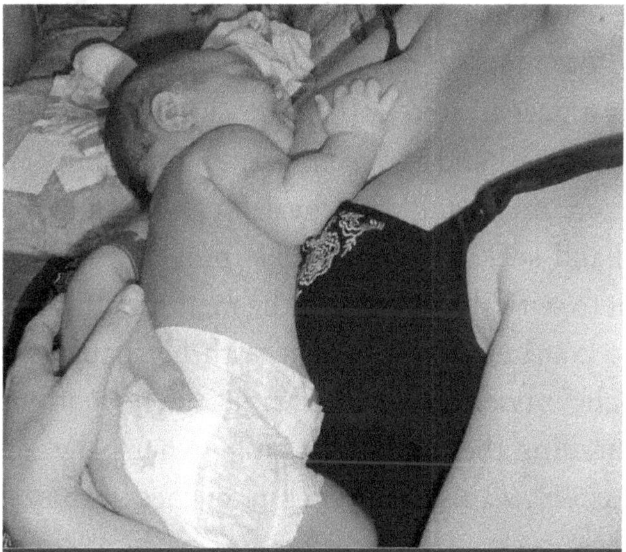

Figure 7. Cheek on breast orients baby and allows her to relax her hands.

Starting with the infant at mom's chest or shoulder (Figure 8a) and allowing him to scan with his cheeks, as in Figure 8b, often results in the baby moving to the breast and self-attaching.

When self-attaching, infants will position their own hands and arms to help identify, move, and shape the nipple area. Mothers are easily convinced that their infants are competent and are using their hands deliberately. Mothers can then be patient and allow their babies time to figure out the best way to attach. If the infant uses tactile searching with the hand to augment oral searching (perhaps because the tongue is slightly restricted and retracts when the mouth opens wide, as in Figure 6b) (note the normal tongue position during latch in Figure 1b), they will usually mouth the hand once it lands on or below the nipple (Figure 9). Educating the mother that this is a normal step in the sequence, and that the baby will move the hand and then re-attempt latching prevents her from interfering with the self-calming and orienting that hand sucking at the nipple provides. Allowing the infant to self-calm helps keep the mother calm and allows her to continue to be patient with her baby as well. If the baby misses the attachment at the next attempt, try encouraging the mother to snuggle her baby's body in more closely so his cheek or chin touches the breast.

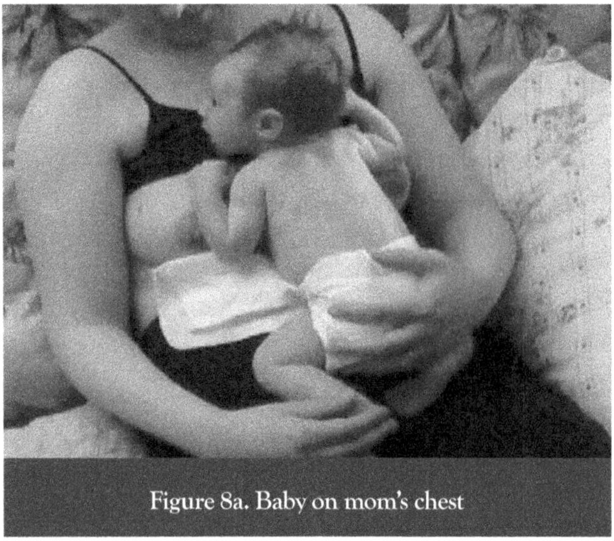

Figure 8a. Baby on mom's chest

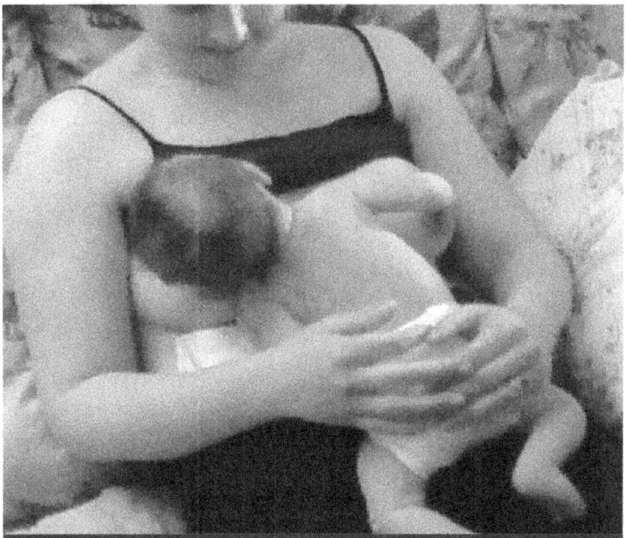

Figure 8b. Scanning for the breast with his cheeks.

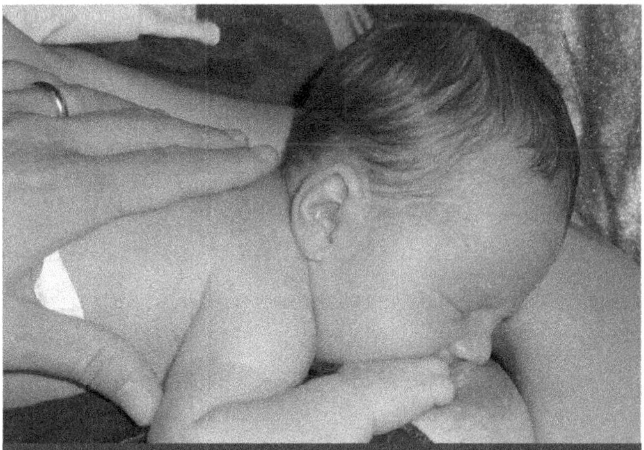

Figure 9. Baby sucking hand placed immediately below the nipple. Once calmed, the baby moves the hand and attaches to the breast in the same place.

If a mother has sore or damaged nipples, you may want to help the mother limit tactile searching, as the baby's grasp response will lead him to pinch or squeeze the nipple with the hand. This can cause pain in damaged nipples. Making sure that the baby's face touches the breast at all times will increase oral searching and decrease tactile searching if the mother is sore.

Mothers who used pain medication in labor may need to be more patient and proactive. Infants exposed to labor analgesia massage the breast for longer before attaching, and are far less likely to suckle after birth. Staff is often concerned about infant blood glucose levels or excessive weight loss. Keeping the baby skin-to-skin with the mother avoids stress-induced rapid utilization of glycogen stores, which reduces the risk of infant hypoglycemia (Christensson et al., 1992; Mazurek et al., 1999). Mothers can be taught to express colostrum onto the nipple for their infant to lick, or into a spoon or small cup for immediate feeding. Babies often latch if returned to the breast right after spoon or cup feeding. These strategies stimulate milk production and provide the infant with calories while he clears the drugs and regains a more normal neurobehavioral status.

Conclusions

Infants actively participate in finding and attaching to the breast. Their participation includes deliberate, but unpracticed, use of their hands to locate, move, and shape the teat.

Maternal and professional understanding of these strategies, and how to work with them, may reduce infant and maternal frustration and improve breastfeeding outcomes

References

Butterworth, G., & Hopkins B. (1988). Hand–mouth coordination in the new-born baby. *British Journal of Developmental Psychology, 6*, 303–314.

Christensson, K., Siles, C., Moreno, L., Belaustequi, A., De la, F. P., Lagercrantz, H., et al. (1992). Temperature, metabolic adaptation and crying in healthy full–term newborns cared for skin-to-skin or in a cot. *Acta Paediatrica, 81*, 488–493.

Colson, S.D., Meek, J.H., & Hawdon, J.M. (2008). Optimal positions for the release of primitive neonatal reflexes stimulating breastfeeding. *Early Human Development, 84*, 441–449.

Lew, A.R., & Butterworth, G. (1995). The effect of hunger on hand-mouth coordination in newborn infants. *Developmental Psychology, 33*, 456–463.

Matthiesen, A.S., Ransjo–Arvidson, A.B., Nissen, E., & Uvnas-Moberg, K. (2001). Postpartum maternal oxytocin release by newborns: Effects of infant hand massage and sucking. *Birth, 28*, 13–19.

Mazurek, T., Mikiel–Kostyra, K., Mazur, J., Wieczorek, P., Radwanska, B., & Pachuta–Wegier, L. (1999). [Influence of immediate newborn care on infant adaptation to the environment]. *Med. Wieku.Rozwol, 3*, 215–224.

Miller, J.L., Sonies, B.C., & Macedonia, C. (2003). Emergence of oropharyngeal, laryngeal and swallowing activity in the developing fetal upper aerodigestive tract: An ultrasound evaluation. *Early Human Development, 71*, 61–87.

Paul, K., Dittrichova, J., & Papousek, H. (1996). Infant feeding behavior: Development in patterns and motivation. *Developmental Psychobiology, 29*, 563–576.

Prechtl, H. F. (1958). The directed head turning response and allied movements of the human baby. *Behaviour, 13*(3/4), 212–242.

Ransjo–Arvidson, A.B., Matthiesen, A.S., Lilja, G., Nissen, E., Widstrom, A.M., & Uvnas–Moberg, K. (2001). Maternal analgesia during labor disturbs newborn behavior: Effects on breastfeeding, temperature, and crying. *Birth, 28*, 5–12.

Smillie, C.M. (2008). How infants learn to feed: A neurobehavioral model. In C.W. Genna (Ed.), *Supporting sucking skills in breastfeeding infants* (pp. 79–95). Sudbury, MA: Jones and Bartlett Publishers.

Sparling, J.W., Van, T.J., & Chescheir, N.C. (1999). Fetal and neonatal hand movement. *Physical Therapy, 79*, 24–39.

van der Meer, A. L., van der Weel, F. R., & Lee, D. N. (1995). The functional significance of arm movements in neonates. *Science, 267*, 693–695.

USLCA

Maternal Intravenous Fluids and Infant Weight

Robin Hirth, BS, MEd, IBCLC, RLC[1]

Tina Weitkamp, MSN, RNC[2]

Alok Dwivedi, PhD, MSc, BSc[3]

Keywords: infant weight loss, maternal IV fluids, labor

Health care providers typically use an infant's weight loss in the first days of life as a measurement of effective feeding. Additional feeding volumes are often recommended when the infant reaches weight loss of 7 to 10 percent of their birth weight. This study examined the relationship of the amount of maternal intravenous fluids (IV) given during labor, and infant maximum weight loss during hospital admission. The method was a retrospective cross-sectional review of medical records for 186 healthy mothers and their infants who delivered at a Baby-Friendly™ certified hospital in southwest Ohio. Maternal average IV mL per hour positively correlated with infant maximum weight loss.

Health care providers typically use an infant's weight loss in the first few days of life as a measurement of effective

1 rlhirth@health-partners.org

2 Tina.Weitkamp@UC.edu

3 Alok_Bhul@yahoo.com

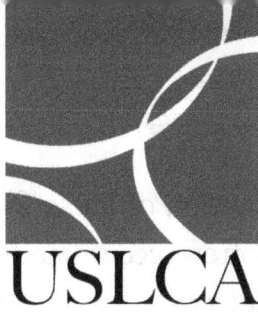

feeding. Supplementation of breastfeeding or increased formula-feeding is often recommended when the infant reaches weight loss of 7 to 10 percent of their birth weight (Academy of Breastfeeding Medicine, 2009; American Academy of Pediatrics, 2005; International Lactation Consultant Association, 2005; Mulder et al., 2010). The range of weight loss can be influenced by a variety of factors. However, minimal research has explored the potential influence of maternal intravenous (IV) volume received during labor.

Influences on Infant Weight Loss after Birth

Increased infant weight loss during the first few days of life in all infants is associated with female gender, epidural, primiparous mother, cesarean section, and feeding method (Martens & Romphf, 2007). Increased infant weight loss in breastfed infants is associated with cesarean section (Saki et al., 2010), delayed onset of lactogenesis (Dewey et al., 2003), suboptimal breastfeeding, exclusive breastfeeding, or breastfeeding with supplements (Chantry et al., 2011; Martens & Romphf, 2007), labor > 14 hours (Dewey et al., 2003), multiparous women who receive labor pain medication (Dewey et al., 2003), and maternal breast variation (Vazirinejad et al., 2009).

Early questions about the effect of the volume of maternal IV fluid and infant weight loss were suggested in articles by Merry and Montgomery (2000) and Dewey et al. (2003). The first study was a master's thesis by Sheehan (2009), which reported that a total maternal intravenous volume of >1225 mL (regardless of duration of fluid intake), cesarean section, and epidural were significant for infant weight loss ≥7% of birth weight at 72 hours of age. Lamp and Macke (2010) studied intrapartum maternal fluid balance (IV fluid administered + oral intake). Infants were weighed at 48 ± 2 hours, and 4.3% were found to have lost ≥ 10%. They found that intrapartum maternal fluid balance was not significant for weight loss. However, type of feed (p= 0.000) and number of wet diapers were significant for weight loss (p= 0.003). Chantry et al. (2011) found that excessive weight loss was independently related to intrapartum fluid balance. The relative risk for excessive weight loss more than tripled with a maternal positive fluid balance exceeding 200 mL/hour when compared to 100 mL/hour.

Noel-Weiss et al. (2011) found that the timing and amounts of fluid (including oral intake and IV fluids) correlated with the output and weight loss of breastfed newborns. The authors observed a 24-hour post-birth period of newborn diuresis and fluid-balance correction. Therefore, they recommended that a newborn weight measurement at 24 hours replace birth weight as baseline for weight change assessment.

Method

Design

The study was a retrospective cross-sectional review of medical records for mother/infant dyads. Mother/infant dyads were excluded for maternal conditions that may impact infant birth weight or weight loss, including maternal fever, diabetes (gestational and type I or II), placental abruption, chronic or pregnancy-induced hypertension, diuretics, fever, oligohydramnios, polyhydramnios, placenta previa, positive screen for drugs of abuse, renal or cardiac disease, rupture of membranes ≥ 24 hours, sexually transmitted infections, and incomplete or inconsistent information.

Mother/infant dyads were excluded for infant conditions that may impact infant birth weight or weight loss, including birth weight < 2500 or > 4000 grams, gestational age < 37 or > 42 weeks, admission to Special Care Nursery, cardiac disease, congenital anomalies, gastrointestinal disease, thick meconium-stained fluid, phototherapy, renal disease, respiratory disease, sepsis, multiple birth, and incomplete or inconsistent information.

Sample

The study population was mothers and their infants who delivered at a Midwestern American hospital. The hospital has been certified continuously as a Baby-Friendly Hospital™ since 2000. Initially, the sample size of 200 mother/infant dyads was chosen to capture 10% of the 2000+ annual births.

Based on the review of literature, it was expected to have 5% to 10% relative change in mean weight loss, with a standard deviation of 2% to 5%. Considering the most conservative estimate of standard deviation as 5 with absolute deviation in mean weight loss as 15% of mean, with 5% level of significance, the estimated minimum sample size was determined to be 174. A total of 518 mother/infant dyads were reviewed during December 2008 and April 2009 until 200 met the study objectives.

Procedures

A data-collection tool was utilized by the study investigators to review electronic and paper medical records, and record maternal demographics, prenatal history, labor and delivery, and IV intake; and infant demographics and weights throughout hospital admission of two-to-four days.

To minimize missing data and increase validity, maternity nursing staff were informed of the study and encouraged to make extra efforts to accurately chart IV volume and start/end times. Unclothed infants were weighed at birth, and on each additional in-patient hospital day during the 12-hour night shift. Digital infant scales were calibrated by the hospital clinical engineering department every two weeks during the study, and all scales remained accurate.

Ethical Considerations and Protection of Human Subjects

The study was approved by the University of Cincinnati Institutional Review Board and the Mercy Hospital Fairfield Medical Staff Quality Committee.

Statistical Analysis

The primary outcome measure was maximum percent weight loss from the birth weight on any subsequent daily weight during hospital stay (2, 3, or 4 days). The quantitative variables are described using mean and standard deviation (SD). Categorical variables are described using frequency and proportions. Non-normal variable, average IV fluid mL/hour, was transformed into log scale to induce normality needed to satisfy for parametric data analysis. Unadjusted ordinary linear regression was used to select important cofactors for multiple ordinary linear regression analysis. All the significant cofactors at 5% level of significance in the univariate analysis were included in multivariable analysis.

Stepwise, multiple linear regression was used to assess factors associated with maximum weight loss with 5% level of entry, and 10% level of stay in the model. First-order interaction effect was explored for some of the important cofactors before finalizing the model. However, no interaction effect was found to be significant. Variables with variance inflation factor more than 10 were considered as collinear.

Model performances were described using R^2 statistics. Univariate results are reported using unadjusted regression coefficient (URC), with their 95% confidence intervals (CI) and adjusted results are reported using adjusted regression coefficient (ARC) with their 95% CI. All the results with less than 5% were considered as significant results. A scatter plot was constructed to show the relationship between IV fluids per hour and maximum infant weight loss (see below).

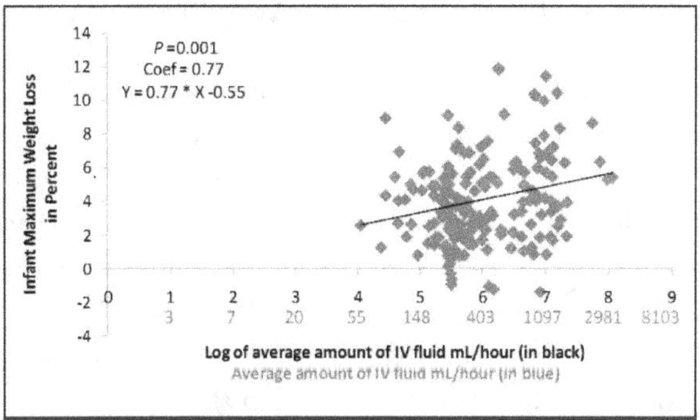

Infant Maximum Weight Loss by mL/Hour

Results

A total of 200 subjects met the inclusion criteria and were included in the study. Out of 200, 14 mothers did not receive IV fluid. Coefficient of variation of subjects who received IV fluid was 57%, and those who did not as 63%. During analysis, the 14 mothers who did not receive any IV fluid were excluded, resulting in $n = 186$. Mean maximum weight loss was 4.08% (SD: 2.57).

Maternal demographics, prenatal history, labor-and-delivery statistics are described in Table 1 [link to Table 1]. In the univariate analysis, mother's age, marital status, ethnicity, insurance status, induction, augmentation, medication use during labor and delivery, anesthesia, method of delivery, feeding method, and IV fluid per hour were found to be significantly associated with maximum weight loss. For every one percent increase in average mL per hour, the infant maximum weight loss percent will increase by 0.0077 (see below).

Example for Infant Maximum Weight Loss Percent

For every one percent increase in average mL per hour, the infant maximum weight-loss percent will increase by 0.0077. For example, assume a 5% infant maximum weight loss, and a change in average IV ml per hour from 150 to 225 (a 50% increase). Then maximum weight-loss percent would be predicted to increase by 0.0077 x 50, which is 0.39, giving a total maximum weight-loss percent of 5.39 (5 + 0.39).

The variance inflation factor was found to be more than 10 for three variables (medication used during labor and delivery, anesthesia, and method of delivery). This indicates that these three variables are highly collinear. Thus, we developed various multivariable regression models after including and excluding collinear variables. After including all collinear variables, in multivariable analysis, race, medications during labor and delivery, and feeding methods, remained significant. These variables explained 46% (R^2=0.46) of the variability in the maximum percent weight loss.

Infants breastfeeding with supplements had significantly less weight loss when compared to those exclusively breastfed after adjusting other significant cofactors. After excluding medications during labor and delivery, anesthesia, and method of delivery, IV fluid was found to be one of the most significant factors associated with maximum weight loss after adjusting for feeding method (Table 1). This model explains 28% of the variability in the maximum weight loss (R^2=0.28).

Discussion

Maternal average IV mL per hour positively correlated with infant maximum weight loss. However, there are many factors related to infant weight loss, and if an infant's weight loss is excessive, then additional assessments are indicated, including, but not limited to:

Maternal Assessment

- Maternal IV fluid during labor
- Stage of lactogenesis
- Risk factors for breastfeeding complications

Infant Assessment

- Confirm current weight loss
- Repeat weight check in 12 to 24 hours
- Evaluate infant feeding frequency and effectiveness
- Evaluate infant hydration status
- Evaluate infant output

Although limited research exists in this area, preliminary results among current studies are trending to include maternal IV fluids in the assessment of an infant's weight loss in the first days of life before ordering supplementation.

Recommendations

Limitations of this study are primarily methodology related. Additional research is needed to confirm correlation between maternal IV fluid and infant weight loss. Enhancements to this study design may include: a) multi-site study to increase external validity, especially including hospitals without Baby-Friendly certification, and with different racial and socioeconomic population; b) prospective method to increase data-collection accuracy; c) reduced exclusion criteria to increase ability to apply to larger populations; d) standardized infant weight checks to 24, 48, 72 hours (±2); and e) increased sample size.

Acknowledgements

This study was supported by an Institutional Clinical and Translational Science Award, NIH/NCRR Grant Number 5UL1RR026314-03. Its contents are solely the responsibility of the authors and do not necessarily represent the official views of the NIH.

The authors would like to thank Linda Baas, Athena Farmer, John (Chuck) Schafer, Rakesh Shukla, and Michele Stokes.

References

Academy of Breastfeeding Medicine. (2009). ABM clinical protocol #3: Hospital guidelines for the use of supplementary feedings in the healthy term breastfed neonate, revised 2009. *Breastfeeding Medicine, 4*(3), 175-182. doi:10.1089/bfm.2009.9991

American Academy of Pediatrics. (2012). Policy statement. Breastfeeding and the use of human milk. *Pediatrics, 129*(3), e827-e841. doi:10.1542/peds.2011-3552

Chantry, C., Nommsen-Rivers, L., Peerson, J., Cohen, R., & Dewey, K. (2011). Excess weight loss in first-born breastfed newborns relates to maternal intrapartum fluid balance. *Pediatrics, 127*(1), e171-e179.

Dewey, K., Nommsen-Rivers, L., Heinig, M., & Cohen, R. (2003). Risk factors for suboptimal infant breastfeeding behavior, delayed onset of lactation, and excess neonatal weight loss. *Pediatrics, 112*(3), 607-619.

International Lactation Consultants Association. (2005). *Clinical guidelines for the establishment of exclusive breastfeeding, 2nd edition.* Raleigh, NC: Author.

Lamp, J., & Macke, J. (2010). Relationships among intrapartum maternal fluid intake, birth type, neonatal output, and neonatal weight loss during the first 48 hours after birth. *JOGNN: Journal of Obstetric, Gynecologic, & Neonatal Nursing, 39*(2), 169-177.

Martens, P., & Romphf, L. (2007). Factors associated with newborn in-hospital weight loss: Comparisons by feeding method, demographics, and birthing procedures. *Journal of Human Lactation, 23*(3), 233-241.

Merry, H., & Montgomery, A. (2000). Do breastfed babies whose mothers have had labor epidurals lose more weight in the first 24 hours of life? *ABM NEWS and VIEWS, 6*(3), 21. Retrieved from http://www.draparrilla.com/pdf/abstracts%20WIC.pdf

Mulder, P., Johnson, T., & Baker, L. (2010). Excessive weight loss in breastfed infants during the postpartum hospitalization. *JOGNN: Journal of Obstetric, Gynecologic, & Neonatal Nursing, 39*(1), 15-26.

Noel-Weiss, J., Woodend, K., Peterson, W., Gibb, W., & Groll, D. (2011). An observational study of associations among maternal fluids during parturition, neonatal output, and breastfed newborn weight loss. *International Breastfeeding Journal, 6*:9. doi:10.1186/1746-4358-6-9

Saki, A., Eshraghian, M., Mohammad, K., Foroushani, A., & Bordbar, M. (2010). A prospective study of the effect of delivery type on neonatal weight gain pattern in exclusively breastfed neonates. *Neonatal Intensive Care, 23*(3), 52-54.

Sheehan, K. (2009). *The role of intrapartum intravenous therapy and method of delivery on newborn weight loss: Challenging the 7% rule.* Master thesis. Retrieved from http://dr.library.brocku.ca/ bitstream/ handle/10464/2925/Brock_Sheehan_Kim_2009. pdf?sequence=1

Vazirinejad, R., Darakhshan, S., Esmaeili, A., & Hadadian, S. (2009). The effect of maternal breast variations on neonatal weight gain in the first seven days of life. *International Breastfeeding Journal,* 4:13. Retrieved from: http://www.internationalbreastfeedingjournal.com/content/4/1/13

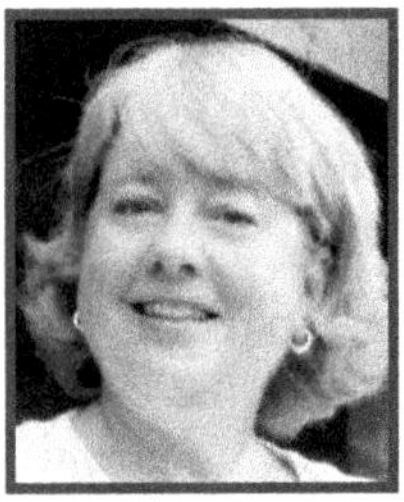

Robin Hirth, MEd, BS, IBCLC, RLC is a board certified lactation consultant with 30 years' experience working with breastfeeding families. She currently works as a lactation consultant at Mercy Health-Fairfield Hospital in the Cincinnati, Ohio area. She planned and implemented the strategic plan, which qualified Mercy Hospital Mt. Airy in Cincinnati for the Baby-Friendly Hospital™ Award in 1997. Her many volunteer efforts include speaking at local, regional, and national conferences; and serving as La Leche League Leader, IBLCE Exam Proctor, and Editorial Review Board Member for *Clinical Lactation* and the *Journal of Human Lactation.*

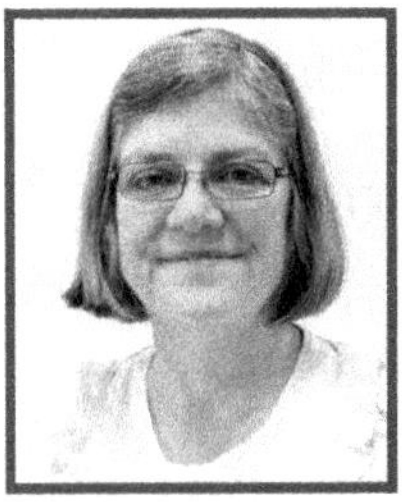

Tina Weitkamp, MSN, RNC is an associate professor of clinical nursing at the University of Cincinnati College of Nursing. She has over 30 years' experience in maternity nursing, including staff nurse, clinical nurse specialist, and clinical instructor. A focus of her teaching has been on newborn and postpartum care, with an interest in breastfeeding. In the past

Ms. Weitkamp has answered questions on breastfeeding for NetWellness.org. Publications, speaking engagements, and international health clinical activities allow her to share her extensive skills and knowledge across the United States to Canada, Tanzania, Honduras, Japan, and Taiwan.

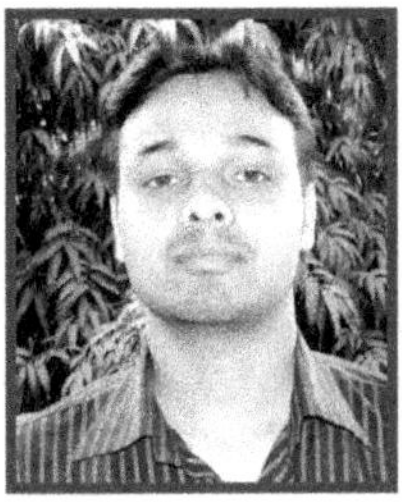

Alok Dwivedi, PhD, M.Sc., B.Sc. is a Post Doctoral Fellow in Biostatistics at the Division of Biostatistics and Epidemiology, Department of Environmental Health, University of Cincinnati (UC). He also works in the Center for Biostatistical Services, UC College of Medicine, and in the Center for Clinical Translation Science and Training at Cincinnati Children's Hospital Medical Center. Dr. Dwivedi has currently accepted an Assistant Professor position in the Division of Biostatistics and Epidemiology, Department of Biomedical Sciences, Texas Tech University Health Sciences Center, El Paso, Texas. His research focuses on count data modeling, skewed data modeling, multilevel modeling, quantile regression, and meta-analysis. He is a member of Editorial Review Board of *Health Journal, SCIRP* and statistical reviewer of *American Heart Journal* and *Circulation.* Dr. Dwivedi also participates in reviewing intramural and methodological proposals.

USLCA

Intrapartum Nurse's Guide to Protecting, Promoting and Supporting Breastfeeding: Another Ten Steps

Martha (Marty) Gibson, PhD, RN, CHES[1]

Betty Carlson Bowles, PhD, RNC, IBCLC, RLC[2]

Lauren Jansen, PhD, RN[3]

Jane Leach, PhD, RNC, IBCLC, RLC[4]

Keywords: breastfeeding, perinatal care, labor & delivery

The intrapartum period is a crucial time for implementing steps to protect, promote, and support breastfeeding. Labor and delivery nurses may be more concerned with the immediate safety of the mother and fetus than with future implications for breastfeeding. The purpose of this article is to review the potential effects that prenatal education and intrapartum practices and interventions have on lactation,

1 Martha.gibson@mwsu.edu
2 Betty.bowles@MWSU.edu
3 Lauren.jansen@mwsu.edu
4 Jane.leach@mwsu.edu

and to encourage nurses to thoughtfully consider these effects in their clinical practices. By implementing these recommendations they can better educate the mother, empower her to make informed choices, avoid unnecessary intrusion into the normal birth process, and maximize the potential for meeting her breastfeeding goals.

The "Ten Steps to Successful Breastfeeding" issued by the World Health Organization (WHO) and the United Nations Children's Fund (UNICEF) (1989) are evidence-based, have endured for over 20 years, and have been the basis for many national and international breastfeeding promotional campaigns. These steps largely exclude the prenatal and intrapartum period, which is a crucial time for implementing steps to protect, promote, and support breastfeeding. Nurses functioning in this often stressful environment may be more concerned with the immediate safety of the mother and fetus than with future implications for breastfeeding. The purpose of this article is to review potential effects intrapartum practices have on lactation, and to encourage nurses to thoughtfully consider these effects in their clinical practices. By implementing these recommendations, nurses can better educate the mother, empower informed choices, avoid unnecessary intrusion into the normal birth process, and maximize the potential for meeting her breastfeeding goals.

Case Study

Mary, pregnant for the first time and eager to breastfeed her first child, presented at term to the Labor and

Delivery (L&D) unit in labor. The nurse's first interventions were to put her to bed, place her on the electronic fetal monitor (EFM), and perform a vaginal exam. She was partially effaced and dilated with an early-labor contraction pattern. When her contractions slowed, her bag of water was broken to augment her labor. Her contractions increased in frequency and intensity, and she was offered an epidural. The epidural precipitated a drop in blood pressure and deceleration of the fetal heart rate (FHR), both of which recovered after the bolus of intravenous (IV) fluid. Because of the FHR deceleration, internal EFM was initiated. After the epidural, her contractions decreased in intensity, and a pitocin augmentation had begun.

She assumed an active-labor pattern, but with slow dilatation and effacement. When the physician came, Mary was told that after a trial of labor with failure to progress, and because her membranes had been ruptured for some time, a cesarean section was recommended to avoid the likelihood of infection. After the cesarean delivery, the baby was taken to the nursery, where he remained for several hours and was given formula due to a low blood sugar. The baby was sleepy and showed no interest in the first breastfeeding.

In spite of regular feedings, Mary's milk was late coming in and she gave supplemental formula after each feeding. Her milk supply continued to decrease, and she quit breastfeeding at 2 weeks. Mary was disappointed and depressed because she had "failed" to achieve her goal of breastfeeding her baby. What perinatal interventions put

Mary at risk for lactation "failure?" What nursing interventions or anticipatory guidance could have protected, promoted, and supported her intention to breastfeed?

Care of the Laboring Mother

The L&D nurse is in a strategic position to assess the mother's knowledge and preparation for labor, birth, and parenting, and to ensure that the mother's wishes and goals are communicated to the rest of the staff. Her role is vital to ensure that informed consent is obtained for the choices the mother will make during this intrapartal period (Lally et al., 2008). Three essential admission assessments related to informed consent are the mother's knowledge of the benefits of breastfeeding and risks of formula feeding; the impact of analgesia and anesthesia on labor, the infant, and the lactation process; and the knowledge of and experience with non-pharmacologic comfort measures to minimize the use and impact of pharmacologic measures. The Academy of Breastfeeding Medicine (ABM) recommends that these topics be included in prenatal education (ABM, 2008).

L&D nurses should collaborate with childbirth educators in their area to ensure continuity of care on these vital issues, which require time for discussion and assimilation, and therefore cannot ideally be initiated upon admission to labor. With such collaboration, the L&D nurse need only to assess the patient's knowledge and preferences in order to ensure informed consent.

Table 1. Another Ten Steps for Intrapartum Nurses
1. Assess the mother's knowledge of the benefits of of breastfeeding and risks of formula feeding to ensure informed consent for feeding choice.
2. Assess the mother's knowledge of the impact analgesia and anesthesia has on labor, the infant, and the lactation process.
3. Assess the mother's knowledge of, experience with, and motivation for the use of non-pharmacologic comfort measures to customize teaching and labor support to avoid or minimize pharmacologic measures.
4. Encourage ambulation for as long as the laboring woman is comfortable.
5. Discourage the recumbent position and suggest frequent position changes for mothers confined to bed.
6. Encourage oral hydration and nourishment, unless contraindicated, and carefully monitor fluid intake and output.
7. Place baby immediately on mother's chest, and leave the baby skin-to-skin to encourage bonding, breast-seeking, and breastfeeding behaviors.
8. Delay routine eye prophylaxis and vitamin K injections until after the first breastfeeding is accomplished.
9. Delay the baby bath until after the first breastfeeding.
10. Initiate breast pumping within the first hour if the infant is transferred to the NICU without the opportunity for skin-to-skin contact and breastfeeding.

If the patient has not participated in a childbirth education program, the nurse is in a position to assess knowledge, and provide as much information to bridge any knowledge gap as the patient's stage of labor and interest allows.

Benefits of Breastfeeding and Risks of Formula-Feeding

The first essential assessment is the mother's knowledge of the benefits of breastfeeding and risks of formula feeding. Breastfeeding decreases the incidence of infant and maternal acute and chronic disease, protects the infant from hazards associated with formula feeding, and significantly decreases the cost of infant feeding and health care (Spatz & Lessen, 2011; Walker, 1992, 1998). The International Lactation Consultant Association (ILCA) states that "routine supplementation represents unnecessary risks to the infant, and is detrimental to a woman's self-confidence and her milk supply" (ILCA, 2000, p.2). The ABM (2010) proposes that all pregnant women be given information on these benefits and risks. Therefore, before ascertaining the mother's preferred method of infant feeding, the L&D nurse should assess the mother's knowledge of benefits of breastfeeding, and risks of formula-feeding, to ensure informed consent.

Whether or not the mother has adequate knowledge, the L&D nurse should maintain the normalcy of breastfeeding by assuming that the mother will breastfeed.

She can explain the protocol of putting the baby skin-to-skin with the mother to be dried and left until after he has breastfed. If the mother says she is not planning to breastfeed, the nurse can inform her that the same procedure will be followed because it is just as important for formula-fed babies to have this skin-to-skin contact. Depending on the mother's stage of labor at admission, and her interest in pursuing the subject, the nurse can provide basic information about some of the many benefits of breastfeeding and the risks of formula.

Labor Analgesia/Anesthesia

Other issues requiring informed choice on admission to labor involve comfort measures and pain management. To make an informed decision mothers must understand the impact of analgesia and anesthesia on labor, the infant, and the lactation process. Maternal analgesia results in lower Infant Breastfeeding Assessment Tool (IBFAT) suckling scores and early weaning (Riordan etal., 2000). Regional anesthesia can cause poor quality contractions and prolonged labor (Leighton & Halpern, 2002), which interferes with the newborn's spontaneous breast-seeking and breastfeeding behaviors (Wiklund et al., 2009), and has a negative effect on breastfeeding (Heaman, 2005).

Babies of mothers who have epidurals are more likely to be supplemented in the hospital (Baumgarder et al., 2003) and stop breastfeeding in the first 24 hours (Torvaldsen et al., 2006). Consent forms for analgesia/anesthesia usually do not describe labor-altering and lactation-altering side effects. Informed consent for pharmacologic pain relief should begin with prenatal education that includes full, unbiased information about these methods (Lowe, 2004). This is another reason for intrapartum nurses to encourage childbirth education and collaborate with childbirth educators. It then falls to L&D nurses to assess the mother's knowledge of the impact analgesia and anesthesia have on labor, the infant, and lactation.

Non-Pharmacologic Comfort Measures

In addition to assessing the mother's knowledge of analgesia and anesthesia, the nurse should ascertain the mother's knowledge of their alternatives. Because labor pain interpretation is so individual, a variety of pain management options should be available (Lowe, 2002). Hodnett (2002) studied satisfaction with the labor experience and noted that pain, pain relief, and medical interventions had minimal influence, while support, communication, information, and involvement with decision making were the main elements of childbirth satisfaction. Since the prepared-childbirth movement of the mid-1900s, women have sought ways to lessen the need for analgesia/anesthesia and their attendant risks. A Cochrane review showed that women who received labor support had shorter labors, less analgesia, more spontaneous births, infants with higher Apgar scores, and more satisfaction with the birth experience than those without labor support (Hodnet et al., 2011).

Labor support is also associated with timely onset of lactogenesis and improved breastfeeding continuation rates (Nommsen-Rivers et al., 2010). Hospital staffing often does not allow continuous labor support to one woman in labor (Green et al., 2007). Labor support has been shown to be more effective when provided by companions who are not part of the hospital staff (Hodnett et al., 2007). When mothers have inadequate information due to lack of prenatal education or preparation, and do not have a labor companion for support, the nurse is challenged to assist the unprepared mother in pain management techniques, which can be very time consuming. Comfort measures that nurses can use or teach to support persons include relaxation, breathing techniques, position changes, massage, hydrotherapy, applications of heat and cold, guided imagery, counter pressure, and massage (Brown et al., 2001; Simkin, 2007).

Childbirth education often fails to provide unbiased information about these techniques (Torres & De Vries, 2009). Hospital-based prenatal classes may be more focused on orienting women to hospital routines rather than informing them of their options (Carlton et al., 2005). Therefore, the L&D nurse should assess the mother's knowledge of, experience with, and motivation for use of non-pharmacologic comfort measures to customize education and labor support to avoid or minimize pharmacologic measures. One way to initiate this assessment is to inquire about childbirth preparation by asking about the mother's plans for labor and how the nurse can best assist her in comfort measures and pain management. This assessment can initiate whatever dialog the mother's labor status will allow.

Labor Practices and Interventions

In addition to the important role in obtaining informed consent, the L&D nurse can advocate for practices that promote normal labor processes. According to Smith (2007, p. 629), "normal birth is the key and foundation to normal breastfeeding." Lamaze International's position paper on promoting, supporting, and protecting normal birth advocates for allowing labor to begin on its own (Amis, 2007), allowing freedom of movement throughout labor (Shilling et al., 2007), providing continuous labor support (Green et al., 2007), avoiding routine interventions (Lothian et al., 2007), allowing spontaneous pushing in upright positions (DiFranco et al., 2007), and keeping mother and infant together with unlimited opportunities for breastfeeding (Crenshaw, 2007).

Kroeger and Smith (2004) proposed that many L&D practices undermine breastfeeding, including bedrest, supine position, limitation of food and drink, induction of labor, analgesics and regional anesthetics, operative vaginal birth, and cesarean delivery. Unfortunately, the first intervention upon admission to an L&D unit is often bedrest and continuous EFM. Bedrest in the recumbent position can decrease the quality of contractions, slow dilatation and effacement, cause maternal hypotension and decreased uteroplacental blood flow, and increase pain necessitating more analgesia/anesthesia (Zwelling, 2010).

Pitocin augmentation to counteract poor-quality contractions can result in more painful contractions (Simpson & Knox, 2009) necessitating additional analgesia/anesthesia, as well as serious complications, such as placental abruption or uterine rupture that increase the risk for emergency cesarean delivery (Thorsel et al., 2011). Prolonged labor, pitocin augmentation, and labor pain medication are all associated with delayed onset of lactogenesis (Dewey et al., 2003).

Amniotomy [artificial rupture of the membranes] to augment poor quality contractions can increase the incidence of prolapsed cord necessitating cesarean delivery (Smyth et al., 2011), and impose a time limitation on the labor due to the risk of infection from prolonged rupture of membranes (Maharaj, 2007). Cesarean section can result in delayed or diminished maternal/infant contact (Chalmers et al., 2010), delayed onset of milk production (Dewey et al., 2003; Scott et al., 2007), and suboptimal breastfeeding practices (Zarnado et al., 2010). Instrumental and surgical birth can exert excess mechanical forces on the infant's head, disrupting bony structures and affecting the nerve and muscle function necessary for nursing (Smith & Kroeger, 2011).

This cascade of potential complications highlights the importance of nursing interventions that advocate for normal labor processes. The nurse can promote freedom of movement by using intermittent auscultation (20 minutes of every hour) versus continuous electronic monitoring (Lothian et al., 2007). Walking and upright positions have been shown to reduce the length of labor (Lawrence et al., 2009). The nurse can encourage walking or slow dancing, or using rocking chairs, birthing balls, or squat bars (Shilling et al., 2007). Showers or tub baths encourage ambulation for as long as the laboring woman is comfortable. For women confined to bed, the intrapartum nurse can do much to discourage the recumbent position, and to assist with frequent position changes, such as side lying, squatting, and hands-and-knees positions to minimize back labor and facilitate normal rotation and descent of the fetal head (DiFranco et al., 2007).

Another common intrapartum routine is administration of IV fluids, and restriction of oral food and fluids. Inadequate hydration in labor may contribute to dysfunctional labor, and possibly cesarean delivery (Garite et al., 2000). Limitation of oral nutrition and fluids during the intrapartum period can lead to fever, hypotension (Eslamian et al., 2006), dehydration, ketosis, hyponatremia, and maternal stress (ShartsHopko, 2010), all of which can negatively affect breastfeeding. O'Sullivan and colleagues (2010) found that eating during labor did not influence obstetric or neonatal outcomes. Over administration of intravenous fluids can cause postpartum edema, which can delay the onset of lactogenesis (Nommsen-Rivers et al., 2010) and lead to difficulties with latch-on and milk expression (Cotterman, 2004). To avoid these negative influences on breastfeeding, the nurse should encourage oral hydration and nourishment, unless contraindicated, and carefully monitor fluid intake and output (Lothian et al., 2007).

Care of the Neonate

Neonatal practices can also profoundly affect the success of breastfeeding. Skin-to-skin contact, and delayed bathing and newborn prophylactic measures, can improve the success of breastfeeding. Close body contact of the mother and infant during this sensitive period helps regulate the newborn's physiological processes and promote breastfeeding behaviors, as well as stimulating the mother's attention to her infant's needs (Winberg, 2005). This contact facilitates breastfeeding (American Academy of Pediatrics [AAP], 2005; ABM, 2009, 2010), and induces long-term positive effects on mother-infant interaction (Bystrova et al., 2009).

A Cochrane review of studies of early skin-to-skin contact found significant positive effects on early breastfeeding including less crying, more stable temperatures, higher blood-glucose levels, and longer breastfeeding duration, as well as improved maternal affectionate behaviors and attachment behaviors (Moore et al., 2007). Because babies placed on their mother's chest make crawling movements toward the breast, root, latch-on, and suck, this contact should be uninterrupted until after the first feeding at the breast (Righard & Alade, 1990). This contact leads to shorter hospital stays (Charpak et al., 2001), and increased duration of breastfeeding (MikielKostyra et al., 2002). The nursing implication is to place the baby immediately on the mother's chest and leave the baby skin-to-skin, allowing ample time to encourage bonding, breast-seeking, and breastfeeding behaviors.

The AAP recommends that drying of the infant, performing initial physical assessment, and Apgar scoring should be done with the baby skin to skin with the mother, and that weighing, measuring, and bathing be delayed until after the first breastfeeding (AAP, 2005). The intrapartum nurse can encourage delay of cord clamping until it stops pulsing, and ensure that other necessary interventions do not interfere with the early, time-sensitive, skin-to-skin contact (Sobel et al., 2011). The administration of prophylactic medications should also be delayed to allow uninterrupted mother/baby contact and breastfeeding (AAP, 2005; ABM, 2010). The baby bath should also be delayed until the first breastfeeding is accomplished.

The nurse can facilitate implementation of these standards, and support the likelihood of a successful first breastfeed, by providing privacy and limiting visitors. If a sick, premature, or low birthweight infant is transferred to the NICU before it has the opportunity for skin-to-skin contact and breastfeeding, the intrapartum nurse can assist the mother to initiate breast pumping within the first hour of birth. This has been shown to increase milk volume and decrease the time to lactogenesis stage II (Parker et al., 2012).

This review of the potential effects intrapartum practices and interventions have on lactation and breastfeeding was intended to encourage intrapartal nurses to thoughtfully consider these effects and implement the recommendations summarized in Table 1 into their clinical practices. By doing so, nurses can support choices made during the prenatal period, better educate the mother, empower her to make informed choices, avoid unnecessary intrusion into the normal birth process, and maximize the potential for meeting her breastfeeding goals.

References

Academy of Breastfeeding Medicine. (2008). ABM clinical protocol #5: Peripartum breastfeeding management for the healthy mother and infant at term. *Breastfeeding Medicine, 3*(2), 129-132.

Academy of Breastfeeding Medicine. (2009). ABM clinical protocol #3: Hospital guidelines for the use of supplementary feedings in the healthy term breastfed neonate. *Breastfeeding Medicine, 4*(3), 175-182.

Academy of Breastfeeding Medicine. (2010). ABM clinical protocol #7: Model breastfeeding policy. *Breastfeeding Medicine, 5*(4), 173177.

American Academy of Pediatrics. (2005). Breastfeeding and the use of human milk. *Pediatrics, 115*(2), 496-506.

Amis, D. (2007). Care practice #1: Labor begins on its own. *Journal of Perinatal Education, 16*(3), 16-20.

Baumgarder, D., Muehl, P., Fischer, M., & Pribbenow, B. (2003). Effect of labor epidural anesthesia on breast-feeding of healthy full-term newborns delivered vaginally. *Journal of the American Board of Family Practice, 16*(1), 7-13.

Brown, S., Douglas, C., & Flood, L. (2001). Women's evaluation of intrapartum non- pharmacological pain relief methods used during labor. *Journal of Perinatal Education, 10*(3), 1-8.

Bystrova, K., Ivanovo, V., Edhborg, M., Matthiesen, A., RansjoArvidson, A, Mukhamedrakhimov, R., Uvnas-Moberg, K., & Widstrom, A. (2009). Early contact versus separation: Effects on mother-infant interaction one year later. *Birth, 36*(2), 97-109.

Carlton, T., Callister, L., & Stoneman, E. (2005). Decision making in laboring women: Ethical issues for perinatal nurses. *Journal of Perinatal & Neonatal Nursing, 19*(2), 145-154.

Chalmers, B., Kaczorowski, J., Darling, E., Heaman, M., Fell, D., O'Brien, B., & Lee, L. (2010). Cesarean and vaginal birth in Canadian women: A comparison of experiences. *Birth, 37*(1), 44-49.

Charpak, N., Ruiz-Pelaex, J.G., Figueroa de, C.Z., & Charpak, Y.A. (2001). A randomized controlled trial of kangaroo mother care: Results of follow-up at 1 year of corrected age. *Pediatrics, 108*, 1072-1079.

Cotterman, J.K. (2004). Reverse pressure softening: A simple tool to prepare areola for easier latching during engorgement. *Journal of Human Lactation, 20*, 227-237.

Crenshaw, J. (2007). Care practice #6: No separation of mother and baby, with unlimited opportunities for breastfeeding. *Journal of Perinatal Education, 16*(3), 39-43.

Dewey, K.H., Nommsen-Rivers, L.A., Heinig, M.J., & Cohen, R.J. (2003). Risk Factors for suboptimal infant breastfeeding behavior, delayed onset of lactation and excess neonatal weight loss. *Pediatrics, 112*, 607-617.

DiFranco, J., Romano, A., & Keen, R. (2007). Care practice #5: Spontaneous pushing in upright or gravity-neutral positions. *Journal of Perinatal Education, 16*(3), 35-38.

Eslamian, L., Marsoosi, V., & Pakneeyat, Y. (2006). Increased intravenous fluid intake and the course of labor in nulliparous women. *International Journal of Gynecology and Obstetrics, 93*(2), 102-105.

Garite, T., Weeks, J., Peters-Phair, K., Pattillo, C., & Brewster, W. (2000). A randomized controlled trial of the effect of increased intravenous hydration on the course of labor in nulliparous women. *American Journal of Obstetrics & Gynecology, 183*(6), 15441548.

Green, J., Amis, D., & Hotelling, B. (2007). Care practice #3: Continuous labor support. *Journal of Perinatal Education, 16*(3), 25-28.

Heaman, M.I. (2005). Epidural analgesia during labor and delivery: Effects on the initiation and continuation of breastfeeding. *Journal of Human Lactation, 21*(1), 305-314.

Hodnett, E. (2002). Pain and women's satisfaction with the experience of childbirth: A systematic review. *American Journal of Obstetrics and Gynecology, 186*, S160-172.

Hodnett, E., Gates, S., Hofmeyr, G., & Sakala, C. (2007). Continuous support for women during childbirth. *Cochrane Database Systematic Review,* 2007 (3):CD003766.

Hodnett, E., Gates, S., Hofmeyr, G., Sakala, C., & Weston, J. (2011). *Continuous support for women during childbirth.* Cochrane Summaries. Retrieved from: http://summaries.cochrane.org/CD003766/continuous-support-forwomen-during-childbirth

International Lactation Consultant Association. (2000). *Position paper on infant feeding.* Retrieved from http://www.ilca.org/ files/resources/ilca_publications/InfantFeedingPP.pdf

Kroeger, M., & Smith, L. (2004). *Impact of birthing practices on breastfeeding: Protecting the mother and baby continuum.* Sudbury, MA: Jones & Bartlett Publishers.

Lally, J., Murtagh, M., Macphail, S., & Thomson, R. (2008). More in hope than expectation: A systematic review of women's expectations and experience of pain relief in labor. *BMC Medicine,* 7:7. Retrieved from: http://www.biomedcentral.com/1741-7015/6/7

Lawrence, A., Lewis, L., Hofmeyr, G., Dowswell, T., & Styles, C. (2009). Maternal positions and mobility during first stage of labour. *Cochrane Database Systematic Review,* Apr 15(2):CD003934.

Leighton, B., & Halpern, S. (2002). The effects of epidural analgesia on labor, maternal, and neonatal outcomes: A systematic review. *American Journal of Obstetrics and Gynecology, 186*(5z), s69-s77.

Lothian, J., Amis, D., & Crenshaw, J. (2007). Care practice #4: No routine interventions. *Journal of Perinatal Education, 16*(3), 29-34.

Lowe, N. (2002). The nature of labor pain. *American Journal of Obstetrics & Gynecology, 186,* S16-S24.

Lowe, N. (2004). Context and process of informed consent for pharmacologic strategies in labor pain care. *Journal of Midwifery and Women's Health, 49*(3), 250-259.g

Maharaj, D. (2007). Puerperal pyrexia: A review. Part I. *Obstetrical and Gynecological Survey, 62*(6), 393-399.

Mikiel-Kostyra, K., Mazur, J., & Boltruszko, I. (2002). Effect of early skin-to-skin contact after delivery on duration of breastfeeding: A prospective cohort study. *Acta Paediatrica, 91*(12), 1301-1306.

Moore, E., Anderson, G., & Bergman, N. (2007). Early skin-toskin contact for mothers and their healthy newborn infants (Review). *Cochrane Database of Systematic Reviews* 2007, Issue 3. Art. No.:CD003519.DOI:10.1002/14651858.CD003519.pub2. Retrieved from: http://apps.who.int/rhl/reviews/CD003519.pdf

Nommsen-Rivers, L., Chantry, C., Peerson, J., Cohen, R., & Dewey, K. (2010). Delayed onset of lactogenesis among first-time mothers is related to maternal obesity and factors associated with ineffective breastfeeding. *American Journal of Clinical Nutrition, 92*(3), 574-584.

Nommson-Rivers, L., Mastergeorge, A., Hansen, R., Cullum, A., & Dewey, K. (2009). Doula care, early breastfeeding outcomes, and breastfeeding status at 6 weeks postpartum among low-income primiparae. *Journal of Obstetrical, Gynecological & Neonatal Nursing, 38*(92), 157-173.

O'Sullivan, G., Liu, B., Hart, D., Seed, P., & Shennan, A. (2009). Effect of food intake during labour on obstetric outcome: randomised controlled trial. *British Medical Journal, 338*, b784. Retrieved from: http://www.bmj.com/highwire/filestream/376813/field_highwire_article_pdf/0.pdf

Parker, L., Sullivan, S., Krueger, C., Kelechi, T., & Mueller, M. (2012). Effect of early breast milk expression on milk volume and timing of lactogenesis stage II among mothers of very low birth weight infants: a pilot study. *Journal of Perinatology, 32*(3), 205-209.

Righard, L., & Alade, M. (1990). Effect of delivery room routines on success of first breast-feed. *Lancet, 335*(8723), 1105-1107.

Riordan, J., Gross, A., Angeron, J., Krumwiede, B., & Melin, J. (2000). The effect of labor relief medication on neonatal suckling and breastfeeding duration. *Journal of Human Lactation, 16*(1), 7-12.

Scott, J., Binns, C., & Oddy, W. (2007). Predictors of delayed lactation. *Maternal & Child Nutrition, 3*(3), 186-193.

Sharts-Hopko, N. (2010). Oral intake during labor: A review of the evidence. *MCN, 11*(5), 197-203.

Shilling, T., Romano, A., & DiFranco, J. (2007). Care practice #2: Freedom of movement throughout labor. *Journal of Perinatal Education, 16*(3), 21-24.

Simkin, P. (2007). *Comfort in labor: How you can help yourself to a normal satisfying childbirth.* Retrieved from www.childbirthconnection.org

Simpson, K., & Knox, G. (2009). Oxytocin as a high-alert medication: Implications for perinatal patient safety. *MCN, 34*(1), 8-15.

Smith, L. (2007). Impact of birthing practices on the breastfeeding dyad. *Journal of Midwifery & Women's Health, 52*(6), 621-630.

Smith, L., & Kroeger, M. (2011). *Impact of birthing practices on breastfeeding, 2nd Ed.* Sudbury, MA: Jones and Bartlett Publishers.

Smyth, R., Aldred, S., & Markham, C. (2011). *Amniotomy for shortening spontaneous labour.* Cochrane Pregnancy and Childbirth Group. Retrieved from: http://onlinelibrary.wiley.com/ doi/10.1002/14651858.CD006167.pub2/

Sobel, H., Silvestre, M., Mantaring, J., Oliveros, Y., & Nyunt-U, S. (2011). Immediate newborn care practices delay thermoregulation and breastfeeding initiation. *Acta Paediatrica, 100*, 1127-1133.

Spatz, D., & Lessen, R. (2011). *Risks of not breastfeeding.* Morrisville, NC: International Lactation Consultants Association.

Thorsel, M., Lyrenas, S., Andolf, E., & Kaijser, M. (2011). Induction of labor and the risk for emergency cesarean section in nulliparous and multiparous women. *Acta Obstetricia et Gynecologica Scandinavica, 90*(10), 1094-1099.

Torres, J., & De Vries, R. (2009). Birthing ethics: What mothers, families, childbirth educators, nurses and physicians should know about the ethics of childbirth. *Journal of Perinatal Education, 18*(1), 12-24.

Torvaldsen, S., Roberts, C.L., Simpson, J.M., Thompson, J.F., & Ellwood, D.A. (2006). Intrapartum epidural analgesia and breastfeeding: A prospective cohort study. *International Breastfeeding Journal, 1*(24), 1-7.

Walker, M. (1992). *Summary of the hazards of infant formula.* Raleigh, NC: International Lactation Consultant Association.

Walker, M. (1998). *Summary of the hazards of infant formula, Part 2.* Raleigh, NC: International Lactation Consultant Association.

Wiklund, I., Norman, M., Uvnas-Moberg, K., Ransio-Avidson, A.B., & Andolf, E. (2009). Epidural analgesia: Breastfeeding success and related factors. *Midwifery, 25*(2), e31-38.

Winberg, L. (2005). Mother and newborn baby: Mutual regulation of physiology and behavior– A selective review. *Developmental Psychobiology, 47*(3), 217-229.

WHO/UNICEF. (1989). *Protecting, promoting and supporting breastfeeding: The special role of maternity services.* Geneva: WHO.

Zarnado, V., Svegliado, G., Cavallin, F., Giustardi, A., Cosmi, E., Litta, P., & Trevisanuto, D. (2010). Elective cesarean delivery: Does it have an effect on breastfeeding? *Birth, 37*(4), 275-279.

Zwelling, E. (2010). Overcoming the challenges: Maternal movement. *American Journal of Maternal/Child Nursing, 35*(2), 72-80.

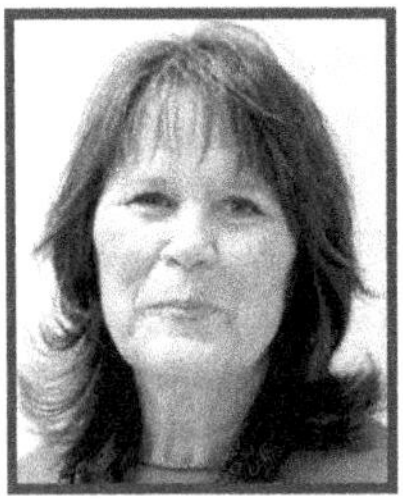

Marty Gibson, PhD, RN, CHES, is Assistant Professor of Nursing at Midwestern State University in Wichita Falls, TX, teaching Community Nursing, Clinical Decision Making, Research and Leadership. She is a Certified Health Education Specialist.

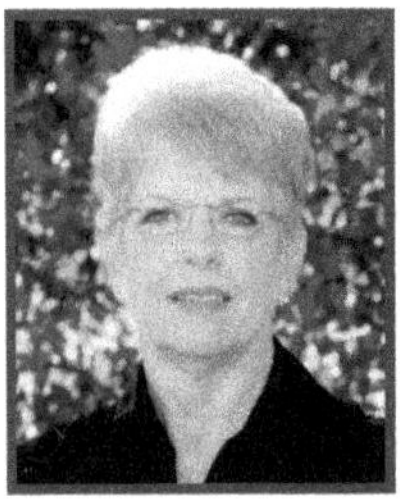

Betty Carlson Bowles, PhD, RNC, IBCLC, RLC, is Assistant Professor of Nursing at Midwestern State University in Wichita Falls, TX, teaching Nursing the Childbearing Family, Community Nursing and Pathophysiology. She is a Childbirth Educator and Lactation Consultant.

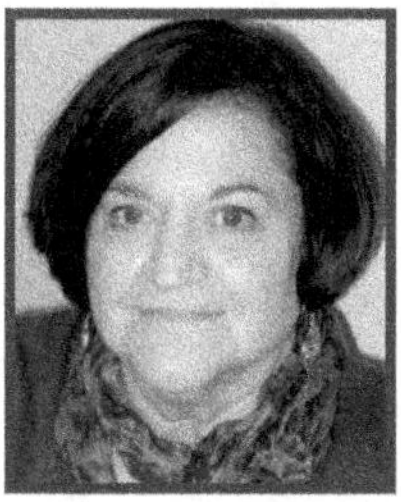

Lauren Jansen, PhD, RN is Assistant Professor of Nursing at Midwestern State University in Wichita Falls, TX, teaching Nursing the Child-bearing Family. She is an obstetrical nurse and childbirth educator.

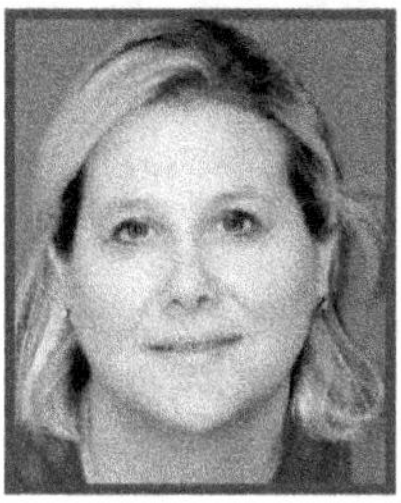

Jane Leach, PhD, RNC, IBCLC, RLC has been a nurse for 30 years, an IBCLC for 20 years and has a certification in maternal-child nursing. She teaches both undergraduate and graduate students and serves as the Coordinator of the Nurse Educator Program at Midwestern State University.

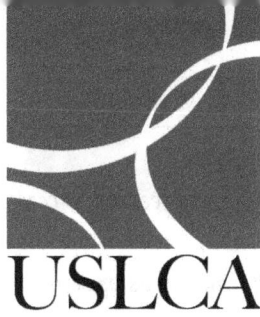

USLCA

Does the Mother's Posture Have a Protective Role to Play During Skin-to-Skin Contact?

Research Observations and Theories

Suzanne Colson, PhD[1]

Keywords: Biological Nurturing, skin-to-skin contact, sudden unexpected postnatal collapse

Skin-to-skin contact during the first hour following birth is the gold standard in breastfeeding. Although consecutive meta-analyses report no adverse effects, a recent review shows an increase in idiopathic sudden unexpected postnatal collapse (SUPC) in healthy term babies identifying three main risk factors: skin-to-skin contact, breastfeeding, and baby lying prone. Concurrently, authoritative visual materials tacitly promote maternal supine postures illustrating the breast crawl, a form of birth skin-to-skin contact. The naked baby lies on top of his or her mother's body, in close ventral contact with torso parallel to the floor—a position strongly associated with sudden infant death. Biological Nurturing (BN) research, the first to examine maternal

1 sdccolson@gmail.com

postural effects on breastfeeding success, suggests that a semireclined maternal position is optimal for breastfeeding initiation. The maternal body slope ensures that the baby lies tilted, a position known to promote oxygenation. The angle of maternal recline, a variable central to BN but hitherto ignored in the skin-to-skin and SUPC literature, is unrelated to dress level. This commentary develops a postural argument to increase understanding of the potential role played by the maternal body slope to reduce the risk of idiopathic SUPC.

Consecutive Cochrane meta-analyses promote early skin-to-skin contact (SSC) as the gold standard in breastfeeding initiation, stating that there are no adverse effects (Anderson, Moore, Hepworth, & Bergman, 2003; Moore, Anderson, & Bergman, 2007; Moore, Anderson, Bergman, & Dowswell, 2012). However, in a recent review, Herlenius and Kuhn (2013) report that some infants have died during early SSC, noting a sharp increase in idiopathic, sudden unexpected postnatal collapse (SUPC) in healthy term babies. Although SUPC is rare, most cases occur during the first 2 postnatal hours with the baby lying prone, breastfeeding in SSC. The mother's posture during these events is ignored.

Experts writing in the mainstream literature, internet photo banks, and social media depict mothers of healthy term infants breastfeeding in SSC in various positions: upright, side-lying, laid-back, and flat-lying (Bergman, 2014; Fotolia, 2014; Smillie, Frantz, & Makelin, 2007; Watson Genna, 2013; YouTube, 2014). However, some of the most widely circulated videos and photos of the breast crawl show mothers lying flat, or almost flat on their backs, and by doing so, tacitly promote a supine position. The United Nations Children's Fund (UNICEF) Breast Crawl video has been widely shown around the world, and was developed to demonstrate that babies are capable of getting to the breast by themselves. As such, it is a useful teaching tool. Unfortunately, those watching it often assume that placing a mother lying supine or almost flat on her back is the best position to use when in early SSC.

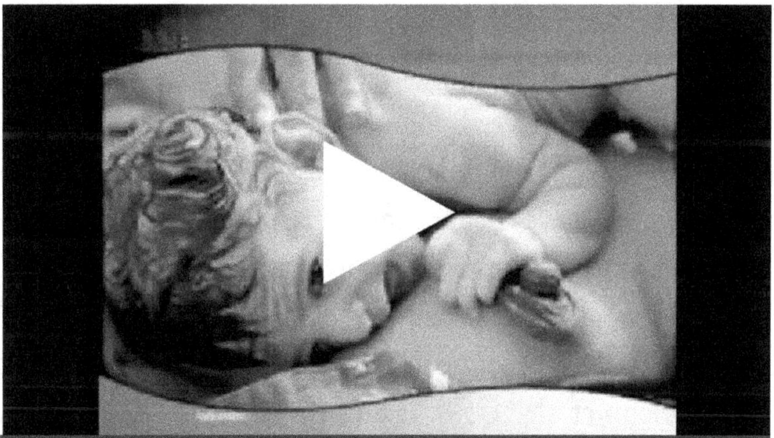

Breast Crawl—Initiation of the Breast Crawl (UNICEF)
http://www.youtube.com/watch?v=YW72pFFEIUo)

The breast crawl is a form of birth SSC thought to aid breastfeeding and self-regulation (Healthy Children Project, 2010, 2012; UNICEF UK Baby Friendly Initiative, 2010; UNICEF/WHO Baby-Friendly USA, 2012; Widström, 2013; Widström, Lilja, AaltomaaMichalias, Dahllöf, Lintula, & Nissen, 2011). In the birth SSC breast crawl, the mother lies supine and the baby is placed prone between the mother's breasts, eyes level with maternal nipples; baby's torso lies flat or horizontal. This position is potentially quite dangerous because it has been strongly associated with sudden infant death (Fleming et al., 1996; Skadberg, Morild, & Markestad, 1998). This prompts a question: does the mother's breastfeeding posture have a protective role to play during SSC?

Is Maternal Posture Protective of Infant Breathing?

Biological Nurturing™ (BN) research is the first to report the impact of maternal posture on breastfeeding success (Colson, 2005a, 2005b, 2006; Colson, Meek, & Hawdon, 2008). For many years, mothers were instructed to initiate breastfeeding sitting upright or lying on their sides, yet BN results, published elsewhere, show that a mean 45° angle of maternal recline is optimal (Colson, 2010a, 2010b, 2012; Colson et al., 2008). Like the birth SSC breast crawl, in BN, the baby also lies prone. But his or her torso is tilted upward; the tilt maintains the baby's head, shoulders and arms elevated, a position noted to increase oxygenation and optimize lung function (Jollye & Summers, 2012; Thoresen, Cowan, & Whitelaw, 1988). BN findings suggest potential drawbacks to placing mothers lying flat, or almost flat, on their backs at any time—especially during the first hours following birth. But so far, researchers studying SSC have not looked at the degree of maternal recline (Moore et al., 2012).

This commentary proposes that maternal posture does make a difference in healthy term infants in the immediate postpartum period, the time when most neonatal SUPC cases occur (Herlenius & Kuhn, 2013). The commentary first summarizes salient aspects of SUPC events, then compares and contrasts the BN mechanisms with the birth SSC breast crawl, and finally makes practice and research recommendations.

Sudden Unexplained Postnatal Collapse

SUPC is an emergency situation, occurring during the first week, characterized by neonatal apnea for 10 seconds, muscle limpness, pallor, bradycardia, cyanosis, collapse, cardiac or respiratory failure, and/or death (Becher, Bhushan, & Lyon, 2012; Poets, Steinfeldt, & Poets, 2011). Herlenius and Kuhn (2013) found such diversity in operational definitions that overall incidence is not comparable. However, national surveys in Germany and Britain, where data for time and neonatal position are available, report 2.6 and 3.5 idiopathic SUPCs per 100,000 live births, respectively; death rates are 1 per 100,000 (Becher et al., 2012; Poets et al., 2011). The authors acknowledge that the incidence is likely underestimated because of restricted time definitions (2 hours), and exclusion of SUPC having rapid and favorable outcomes.

Herlenius and Kuhn (2013) found that roughly half of the SUPC case studies identify the baby's position at the time of the event, and 74% of these are associated with baby prone, skin-to-skin, and cobedding. Typically, a first-time mother and her baby appear healthy and infection free; the baby, born 35 gestational weeks, with APGAR scores of 8 at 5 minutes, and 10 at 10 minutes, is placed prone by the birth attendant, skin to skin. The mother is alone or with the baby's father in the delivery room, initiating breastfeeding. The mother may doze, but awake or asleep, she may not recognize that the baby has collapsed. If the baby dies, the cause, where there is no underlying pathology or other explanation, is "presumed accidental suffocation." See Figure 1.

In view of documented benefits, a professional consensus continues to promote SSC except in cases of maternal sedation, sepsis, extreme fatigue, and lack of continuous professional supervision (Becher et al., 2012; Herlenius & Kuhn, 2013; Poets et al., 2011). These recommendations, although sensitive, fail to consider the role played by the angle of maternal recline, a variable central to BN.

Biological Nurturing and Maternal Recline

BN, a new, mother-centered approach, aims to increase breastfeeding continuance (Colson, 2010a, 2010b, 2012; Colson et al., 2008). BN shares much of the rationale supporting SSC, but interpretations are different; the BN mechanisms are independent of dress level. See Figure 2. In BN, the mother sits semi-reclined—her torso angled from approximately 80° to 35° from the floor. Even a slight recline increases the dimensions from sternal notch to pubes, thus augmenting the amount of maternal body space available to the neonate. Brushing movements release some 20 primitive neonatal reflexes, promoting latch and milk transfer.

Figure 1. Unrecognized Postnatal Collapse

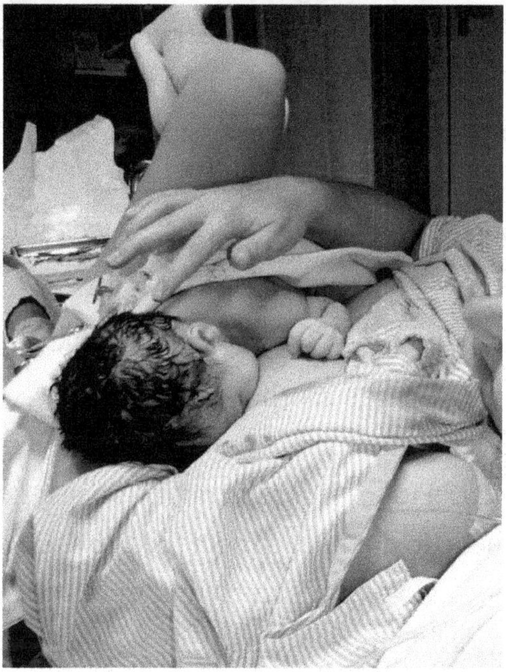

Photo reprinted with courtesy of Professor Berger, Swiss Society of Neonatology, www.neonet.ch, on behalf of the parents. Photograph taken by the father.

The Role of Primitive Neonatal Reflexes

"Primitive neonatal reflexes" is a collective term for inborn reactions, responses, and reflexes (Touwen, 1984). Endogenous and external stimuli release the reflexes, not intention, behavioral state, or dress level (André-Thomas,

Chesni, & Saint-Anne Dargassies, 1960; Brazelton & Nugent, 1995; Colson, 2006, 2010a, 2010b; Colson et al., 2008; Dubowitz, Dubowitz, & Mercuri, 1997; Prechtl, 1977). Offering an alternative interpretation to SSC, the BN mechanisms explain how the SSC breast crawl works: the baby's thighs, calves, feet tops, and soles brush against the mother's body, triggering such reflexes as plantar grasping, the Babinski response, placing, stepping, head bobbing, finger flexion/extension, and rooting as the baby pushes up to locate the breast. Simple reflexes combine to aid locomotion, for example, arm and leg cycling or placing and stepping (Colson, 2006, 2010a, 2010b; Colson et al., 2008).

There are other similarities. In both BN and the birth SSC breast crawl, the mother's hands are free; her body supported; her muscles soft; and both shoulders balanced, not hunched. Furthermore, gravity keeps the baby in place; mothers do not have to hold the baby's back, head, or neck. Gravity also reduces the strength of reflex response, smoothing jerky movements and aiding their expression as latching stimulants. One could argue, supported by compelling birth SSC breast crawl DVDs (Righard & Frantz, 1992; Stark, 2011; Widström, 1996), that supine postures are optimal for breastfeeding initiation, opening the maternal torso dimensions maximally. The science for this argument comes from landmark studies, conducted during the first hour following birth, examining effects of early mother-baby contact for healthy term infants (De Chateau & Wiberg, 1977; Righard & Alade, 1990; Widström,

1988; Widström et al., 1987; Widström et al., 1990). These researchers appear to be the first to illustrate their methods of data collection with photos of breastfeeding mothers lying supine. One objective was to discover if human babies, like other mammals, have species-specific approaching and searching behaviors. Widström (1988, p. 9) and Righard and Alade (1990) asked mothers not to help or "not to push the baby to suck." Results showed that babies crawl unaided to the breast, self-attaching on an average of 55 minutes postbirth. Interestingly, as early as 1988, Widström questioned whether "it might be tiring and even frustrating for the infant to have to crawl to the breast . . . " (p. 29).

We owe Widström and Righard and their colleagues a great debt of thanks for highlighting neonatal competence. Their pioneering SSC studies have much to commend, changing labor ward practices across the world: delaying or eliminating interventions, such as gastric suctioning, that traditionally separated mothers and babies during the first postnatal hour. However, current research methods continue to restrict maternal assistance.

In 2011, Widström et al. described nine sequential innate behaviors priming neonatal self-attachment during the birth SSC breast crawl; they asked 28 participating mothers not to shift their baby's position.

Results reveal that less than two thirds of the babies reached the areola (the primary outcome measure); of those who did, 3 did not suck; and it took up to 45 minutes

Figure 2. Biological Nurturing Independent of Dress State

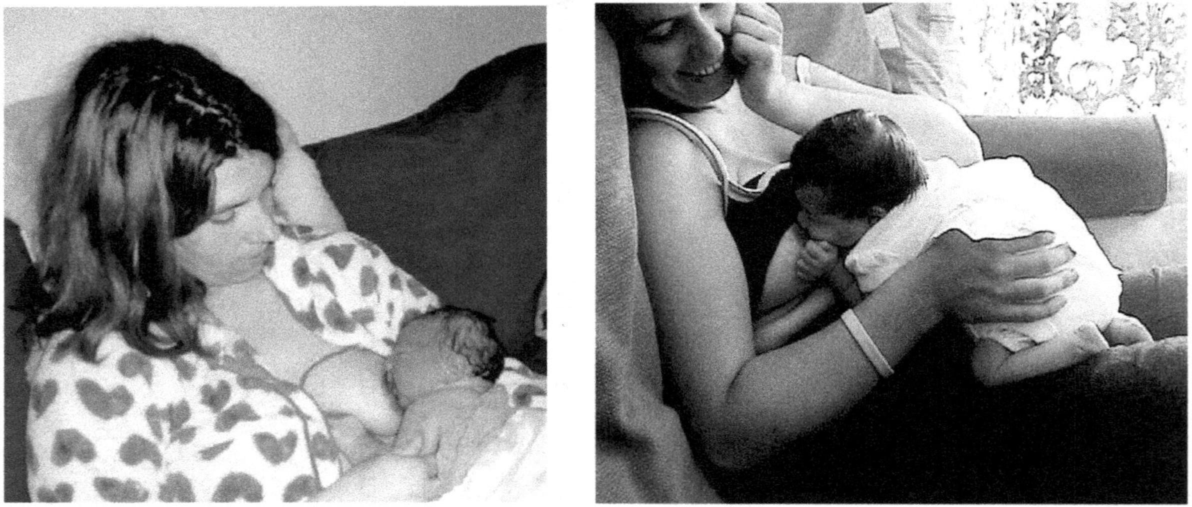

The mother's body slope may help protect neonatal breathing. Left side: First postnatal hour; mother and baby in biological nurturing and skin-to-skin contact. Right side: First postnatal day; mother and baby lightly dressed in biological nurturing.

for others to self-attach, extending the time of SSC to 2 hours. Widström et al. (2011, p. 83) insisted that mothers refrain from physically helping their babies who "work hard and need rests," concluding that babies should stay skin to skin for the first hours following birth, or until the baby accomplishes the nine behavioral stages culminating in self-attachment and/or sleeps.

Placing the onus for first suckling entirely on the baby disregards neonatal fuel economy at the time of cardiorespiratory transition. The birth SSC breast crawl, now suggested for inclusion in lactation management curricula (Widström, 2013), may place undue stress on the baby. The conclusions drawn by Widström et al. (2011; Widström, 2013) must be viewed with extreme caution, considering that so many idiopathic SUPCs for healthy term infants occur during the first 2 hours.

Maybe the question Widström asked in 1988 was justified.

BN research offers different interpretations. Findings suggest that human mothers, unlike lower mammals, participate spontaneously, unless they are told not to. Mothers appear as competent as their babies, often taking the lead. With both hands free, they instinctively place the baby, somewhere on the frontal body space, wherever it feels right; they adjust positions, stroke, groom, check temperature and breathing, shape their breasts, and, occasionally, physically latch the baby without "pushing" (Colson, 2006, 2008a, 2010a, 2010b; Colson et al., 2008).

Although there is some evidence suggesting that neonatal self-attachment reduces nipple sucking (Righard & Alade, 1990; Widström, 2013), the effects of maternal factors, such as posture or spontaneous behaviors stimulating the baby's self-attachment, have not been studied. Clinical and research observations suggest that without instruction, mothers often compulsively protect and help, and this appears to reduce latching time.

A quick birth is known to be a safe birth, and Diaz, Schwarcz, Fescina, and Caldeyro-Barcia (1978) report how vertical maternal postures together with spontaneous pushing and breathing (compared to taught techniques) significantly shorten labor duration. Although there are strong physiological links between birth and lactation (Odent, 1992), it is unknown if such variables as maternal posture and duration of spontaneous newborn searching and finding behaviors promote safety in the breastfeeding context. No research has examined how maternal posture might affect time to first suckling or if a quick latch is safer. Apart from the aforementioned SSC studies, where mothers are placed supine, few have looked at latching times. In the BN sample, raw data show that all 40 mothers participated spontaneously and 2 were in SSC; the mean time to sustained latch was 5 minutes (range 8 seconds to 16 minutes), and, prompted by their mothers, over half the babies self-attached. Latching technique was not routinely assessed; however, breastfeeding duration was 100% at hospital discharge and 100% (87.5% exclusive) at 6 weeks (Colson et al., 2008).

When episodes were filmed during the first postnatal month, these times concur with Bullough, Msuku, and Karonde (1989), who looked at effects of early suckling on postpartum hemorrhage. They calculated a mean time of 7.25 minutes (range 3.5–15 minutes) from birth to first suckling for a sample of 76 babies with spontaneous vertex deliveries who were dried, wrapped, and put to breast within 3 minutes. Without being shown how, mothers repeatedly elicited suckling until baby latched. Taken together, these results suggest that when both mother and baby are allowed to participate spontaneously, latching times may be greatly reduced and relatively stable during the first month. Importantly, maternal spontaneity is not learned behavior; rather, it appears to be released by positions facilitating eye-to-eye contact.

Facilitated eye contact is at the heart of BN. The mother's semi-reclined body slope places her baby's face 8-12 inches from her face, the ideal distance to optimize neonatal visual acuity (Dubowitz, Dubowitz, & Morante, 1980; Klaus & Klaus, 1985). This BN variation of the enface gaze (Klaus & Kennell, 1976) synchronizes eye-to-eye contact, resulting in an intimate, reciprocal, sensorial conversation (Colson, 2010a). Winberg (1995) suggests that mutual stimulation may increase the release of peptide hormones, such as oxytocin, having behavioral effects.

Table 1. Practice Recommendations to Reduce the Incidence of Idiopathic Sudden Unexpected Postnatal Collapse for Healthy Mothers and Healthy Term Babies

Prenatal Education	For Healthcare Providers
	1. Introduce the need to reduce mother-baby separation at birth, delaying routine procedures such as weighing, dressing the baby, eye care, and gastric suctioning. 2. Differentiate BN from SSC and give mothers a choice. 3. Encourage mothers to participate spontaneously during breastfeeding (like they do during birth). 4. Discuss the following: • A range of laid-back maternal breastfeeding postures where comfort is the priority • How the BN angle of recline influences eye-to-eye contact facilitating baby gazing • How mothers naturally protect their baby's breathing, sleep, temperature, and so forth • Inborn protective neonatal reflexes • How babies often latch on in light sleep and drowsy states • That mothers need to be in awake states when they are in SSC or breastfeeding (highlight that the drowsy state for the mother is an "awake" state) 5. Show photos or DVDs of mothers interacting with their babies, that is, placing babies up their bodies, shaping their breasts, helping babies latch when needed and when the baby is in light sleep and drowsy states in SSC and lightly dressed. 6. Promote maternal breastfeeding enjoyment showing mothers who are laughing, stroking, and nurturing. 7. Discourage the use of mobile phones and texting during birth and the first postnatal hours. 8. Discuss safe sleep factors and neonatal back-to-sleep positions.
Immediate Postpartum	**For Doctors, Nurses, Midwives, Doulas, LCs Attending Birth**
	1. Promote BN in SSC, ensuring that every part of the mother's body is supported and that she does not lie supine.

	2. Ensure that the angle of maternal recline facilitates eye-to-eye contact. 3. Replace knitted bulky baby hats or towels that might block eye-to-eye contact with slim cotton baby bonnets and prewarmed cotton-receiving blankets for baby's back warmth. 4. Encourage the mother to participate, giving her permission to help her baby suckle as she feels necessary.
Immediate Postpartum	For Doctors, Nurses, Midwives, Doulas, IBCLCs Attending Birth
	1. Protect the mother's privacy and promote an environment conducive to high oxytocin pulsatility; assess maternal hormonal complexion: comfort, body support, and reactions to the baby and/or people present. 2. Make discrete clinical observations: Ensure constant thermoneutral environment, assessing temperature, and pulse through touch. Assess color and respirations through chest movement. 3. If obstetric needs to lie supine, or if the mother is under the influence of labor analgesics, sedatives or exhausted, or if alone or if it's her first baby, designate one professional person responsible (midwife, doula) for ongoing one-to-one professional supervision, using continuous, but discrete and unobtrusive, at a glance assessments of clinical mother–baby well-being, ensuring patency of neonatal airway. 4. If the mother is awake, aware, and understands her protective role, assure continuity of knowledgeable presence (doula or the baby's father) during the time of cardiovascular transition. 5. Detect as soon as possible any deviation from normal with pediatric referral.
Hospital Discharge	
	1. Review (through purposeful conversation) how the angle of maternal recline may influence inborn mother-baby protective and breastfeeding behaviors. 2. Review and give pamphlet on safe sleeping (positions and other factors).

Gazing, or just thinking about the baby, is recognized to increase oxytocin pulsatility (McNeilly, Robinson, Houston, & Howie, 1983; Riordan, 2010). In turn, this may contribute to the energy economy of both mother and infant (Uvnäs-Moberg, 1989; Winberg, 1995). The key words are mutual and reciprocal. Videos of BN (Colson, 2008a, 2009; Colson, Frantz, & Mohrbacher, 2011) illustrate how the semi-reclined maternal postures promote mother-baby visual interactions, where mothers' facial features, suggest of high oxytocin pulsatility. The BN perspective encourages health care providers to adjust the birthing environment to promote this "oxytocin hormonal complexion" as a key factor, releasing those spontaneous maternal breastfeeding and protective behaviors described earlier (Colson, 2008b, 2010a, 2010b).

Mothers' Position and Infants' Protective Reflex Behaviors

The baby is also born with protective reflex behaviors and two safeguard breathing: spontaneous head lifting and a variation of head righting (Colson, 2006, 2008a, 2010a, 2013a, 2013b). Although sleep states reduce the strength of response (Brazelton & Nugent, 1995; Colson, 2006, 2010a, 2013a, 2013b; Prechtl, 1977), the maternal body slope is a constant impetus, a precious, human species-specific niche aiding the newborn, asleep or awake, skin to skin, or lightly dressed, to release these antigravity movements when needed. Like blinking protects the eyes, and sneezing clears the nostrils, these two defensive reflexes are inborn and independent of dress level. They either protect the neonatal airway, or signal the mother requesting help.

Observe the dynamics in Figure 1. Although mother and baby are in direct ventral SSC, see how the mother's torso is almost horizontal. Her legs in stirrups, she awaits suturing; the angle of her baby's torso mirrors her degree of recline. These semi-flat positions may adversely affect the expression of the baby's protective antigravity reflexes; the degree to which the baby must lift or turn his or her head is steep. At birth, the neck muscles of many infants are not able to counteract strong gravitational pull. Even healthy term babies may struggle, and then be overcome by threatening environmental stimuli; for example, the blockage of the nasal passages by bed clothes or a part of the mother's body.

Figure 1 also shows how gravity works against the mother, blunting her spontaneous reactions. When lying almost flat, maternal mobility appears impaired; placing the baby up her body becomes a monumental task as the blood drains from her arms and hands resisting gravity; her finger tips, identified by Klaus, Kennel, Plumb, and Zuehike (1970) as primary sensorial exploratory organs, become desensitized (M. Bendig, personal communication, June 6, 2010), and her upper limbs tired; mothers often look or act helpless (Colson, 2010a, 2013a).

Furthermore, supine mothers often strain their necks and trapezius muscles when they lift their heads, against gravity, to gaze at their babies. This hampers eye-to-eye contact and may decrease oxytocin pulsatility; mothers, feeling exhausted or bored, may shut out external stimuli or sleep. Together, these observations suggest that visibility in supine postures is not sufficient to release inborn maternal protective behaviors. Even awake, while lying supine or nearly flat, mothers may not be able to see the baby's reflex cues, or if his or her nostrils are obstructed. This offers an alternative explanation for the medical observations that first-time mothers do not notice that their baby has collapsed (Becher et al. 2012; Herlenius & Kuhn, 2013; Poets et al., 2011). During the birth skin-to-skin breast crawl, mothers are simply not in a position to do so.

These observations call into question the exclusion of maternal posture from the birth SSC breast crawl intervention, and the risk factors for SUPC. The American Academy of Pediatrics (2012) recommends keeping healthy newborns in direct SSC until they breastfeed. Bramson et al. (2010) recommend SSC for at least 2 of the first 3 hours following birth. Such guidance needs to be revised to include the potential role played by the angle of maternal recline. BN brings together many factors which may protect neonatal safety, and health care providers should introduce BN during prenatal education, encouraging mothers to participate spontaneously during breastfeeding like they do during birth. Building on recent risk management strategies (Becher et al., 2012; Fleming, 2012; Goldsmith, 2013; Herlenius & Kuhn, 2013; Poets et al., 2011), health professionals should undertake or allocate discrete postpartum assessments to the baby's father or a doula, ensuring that mothers do not lie supine while in SSC or breastfeeding and that their posture optimizes mother-baby eye-to-eye contact (see Table 1 for detailed practice recommendations). Assessments for any mother placed supine for obstetric reasons should be continuous, ensuring professional one-to-one recovery care. Together, these simple measures may help reduce the incidence of rare, but serious, idiopathic SUPC events.

Conclusions

It is well known that a picture is worth a thousand words, and the tacit message conveyed by visual media illustrating the birth SSC breast crawl suggests that a maternal supine posture is the "natural" mammalian way to initiate breastfeeding (Healthy Children Project, 2010, 2012; UNICEF UK Baby Friendly Initiative, 2010; UNICEF/WHO Baby Friendly USA, 2012; Widström, 2013). In Britain, for example, the UNICEF UK Baby-Friendly Initiative (2010) promotes SSC with a photo of a mother lying flat on her back. Although no cause-and-effect relationships can be drawn without further research, it is of note that Becher et al. (2012) report that five healthy term infants died in Britain in 2009-2010 of accidental suffocation during breastfeeding or SSC. These theories and speculations will likely provoke heated discussion; however, the issues can only be resolved through research. Randomized controlled trials should compare BN in SSC and BN when mothers and babies are lightly dressed with the birth SSC breast crawl as standard care, evaluating time to first suckling and spontaneous mother-baby latching techniques to discover if SSC is the independent variable in the birth SSC breast crawl and how the angle of maternal recline affects important variables, such as self-attachment, baby's temperature, blood glucose concentrations, and other physiological variables, as well as bonding and breastfeeding outcomes.

SSC is undoubtedly a lovely way to greet the baby at birth; although linked to SUPC, in fact, SSC may not be a safety factor. The mother's breastfeeding posture may play an important role. Regardless of dress state, the risk may be associated with the angle of maternal recline. While awaiting further research evidence, nothing prevents introducing BN into the SSC equation, auditing effects. If a maternal body slope promotes a neonatal body tilt that protects breathing, mothers and babies may have everything to gain and certainly nothing to lose.

References

American Academy of Pediatrics. (2012). Breastfeeding and the use of human milk: Policy statement. *Pediatrics, 115*, 496–506.

Anderson, G. C., Moore, E., Hepworth, J., & Bergman, N. (2003). Early skin-to-skin contact for mothers and their healthy newborn infants. *Cochrane Database of Systematic Reviews*, (2), CD003519.

André-Thomas, J. M., Chesni, Y., & Saint-Anne Dargassies, S. (1960). *The neurological examination of the infant.* London, United Kingdom: The Medical Advisory Committee of the National Spastic Society.

Becher, J. C., Bhush an, S. S., & Lyon, A. J. (2012). Unexpected collapse in apparently healthy newborns—A prospective national study of a missing cohort of neonatal deaths and near-death events. *Archives of Diseases of Childhood: Fetal and Neonatal Edition, 97*, F30–F34. http://fn.bmj.com/content/97/1/F30.long

Bergman, N. (2014). *Kangaroo mother care: Skin-to-skin contact is also for full term babies.* Retrieved from http://www.kangaroomothercare .com/for-full-term-babies.aspx

Bramson, L., Lee, J. W., Moore, E., Montgomery, S., Neish, C., & Bahjri, K. (2010). Effect of early skin-to-skin mother-infant contact during the first 3 hours following birth on exclusive breastfeeding during the maternity hospital stay. *Journal of Human Lactation, 26*(2), 130–137.

Brazelton, T. B., & Nugent, J. K. (1995). *Neonatal behavioral assessment scale* (3rd ed.). London, United Kingdom: MacKeith Press.

Bullough, C. H. W., Msuku, R. S., & Karonde, L. (1989). Early suckling and postpartum haemorrhage: Controlled trial in deliveries by traditional birth attendants. *The Lancet, 9*, 522–525.

Colson, S. (2005a). Maternal breastfeeding positions: Have we got it right? *The Practising Midwife, 8*(10), 24–27.

Colson, S. (2005b). Maternal breastfeeding positions: Have we got it right? (2). *The Practising Midwife, 8*(11), 29–32.

Colson, S. (2006). *The mechanisms of biological nurturing* Doctoral thesis, Canterbury Christ Church University, Canterbury, England.

Colson, S. (2008a). *Biological nurturing—laid-back breastfeeding* [DVD]. Hythe, England: The Nurturing Project. Available from http://www.biologicalnurturing.com

Colson, S. (2008b). Bringing nature to the fore. *The Practising Midwife, 11*(11), 14–19.

Colson, S. (2009). *Of love and milk* [DVD]. Hythe, England: The Nurturing Project. Available from http://www .biologicalnurturing.com

Colson, S. (2010a). *An introduction to biological nurturing: New angles on breastfeeding.* Amarillo, TX: Hale Publishing.

Colson, S. (2010b). What happens to breastfeeding when mothers lie back? *Clinical Lactation, 1*(1), 11–14.

Colson, S. (2012). Biological nurturing: The laid-back breastfeeding revolution. *Midwifery Today 101*, 9–11, 66. Retrieved from http://www.midwiferytoday.com/articles/biologicalnurturing.asp

Colson, S. (2013a). *Foundations of biological nurturing* [6 twohour webinars]. Morrisville, NC: United States Lactation Consultation Association. Available from http://uslca.org /education-resources/recorded-webinars

Colson, S. (2013b). *Womb to World* [2 webinars] Morrisville, NC: Praeclarus Press. Available from http://PraeclarusPress.com

Colson, S., Frantz, K., & Mohrbacher, N. (2011). *Biological nurturing: Laid-back breastfeeding for mothers* [DVD]. Pasadena, CA: Geddes Productions. Available from http://www.geddesproduction.com

Colson, S. D., Meek, J., & Hawdon, J. M. (2008). Optimal positions for the release of primitive neonatal reflexes stimulating breastfeeding. *Early Human Development, 84*(7), 441–449.

De Chateau, P., & Wiberg, B. (1977). Long-term effect on mother-infant behaviour of extra contact during the first hour postpartum. I. First observations at 36 hours. *Acta Paediatrica Scandinavica, 66*, 137–143.

Diaz, A. G., Schwarcz, R., Fescina, R., & Caldeyro-Barcia, R. (1978). Efectos de la posición vertical materna sobre la evolución del parto. *Clinical Investigative Gynaecology Obstetrics* (Barcelona, Espana), *5*, 101–109.

Dubowitz, L., Dubowitz, V., & Mercuri, E. (1997). *The neurological assessment of the preterm and the full term newborn infant clinics in developmental medicine no. 79*. Philadelphia, PA: Spastics International Medical Publications/JB Lippincott.

Dubowitz, L. M., Dubowitz, V., & Morante, A. (1980). Visual function in the preterm and full term newborn infant. *Developmental Medicine & Child Neurology, 22*, 465–475.

Fleming, P. J. (2012). Unexpected collapse of apparently healthy newborn infants: The benefits and potential risks of skin-to-skin contact. *Archives of Diseases of Childhood, 97*, F2–F3.

Fleming, P. J., Blair, P. S., Bacon, C., Bensley, D., Smith, I., Taylor, E., . . . Tripp, J. (1996). Environment of infants during sleep and risk of the sudden infant death syndrome: Results of 1993-5 case-control study for confidential inquiry into stillbirths and deaths in infancy. Confidential enquiry into stillbirths and deaths regional coordinators and researchers. *British Medical Journal, 313*, 191–195.

Fotolia. (2014). *Royalty Free Stock Photos.* Available at http://www.fotolia.com

Goldsmith, J. P. (2013). Hospitals should balance skin-to-skin contact with safe sleep policies. Pediatricians and the Law. *American Academy of Pediatrics News.* 34:22. http://dx.doi.org/10.1542/aapnews20133411-22

Healthy Children's Center for Breastfeeding Preview. (2010). *The magical hour* [DVD]. Available from http://www.youtube.com/watch?v=pfNUkcxJyhI

Healthy Children Project. (2012). *Healthy children's center for breastfeeding.* Retrieved from http://www.healthychildren.cc /skin2skin.htm

Herlenius, E., & Kuhn, P. (2013). Sudden unexpected postnatal collapse of newborn infants: A review of cases, definitions, risks and preventive measures. *Translational Stroke Research,* 4(2), 236–247. http://www.ncbi.nlm.nih.gov/pmc/articles/ PMC3599160/

Klaus, M. H., & Kennell, J. H. (1976). *Maternal-infant bonding.* St Louis, MO: Mosby.

Klaus, M. H., Kennell, J. H., Plumb, N., & Zuehike, S. (1970). Human maternal behaviour at the first contact with her young. *Pediatrics,* 46(2), 187–192.

Klaus, M. H., & Klaus, P. H. (1985). *The amazing newborn.* Reading, MA: Addison-Wesley Publishing Company, Inc.

Jollye, S., & Summers, D. (2012). *Management of respiratory disorders.* In Boxwell, G. (Ed.), Neonatal intensive care nursing, (2nd ed.). New York, NY: Routledge.

McNeilly, A. S., Robinson, I. C. A., Houston, M. J., & Howie, P. W. (1983). Release of oxytocin and prolactin in response to suckling. *British Medical Journal, 286,* 257–259.

Moore, E. R., Anderson, G. C., & Bergman, N. (2007). Early skinto-skin contact for mothers and their healthy newborn infants. *Cochrane Database of Systematic Review,* (3), CD003519.

Moore, E. R., Anderson, G., Bergman, N., & Dowswell, T. (2012). Early skin-to-skin contact for mothers and their healthy newborn infants. *Cochrane Database of Systematic Review,* (5), CD003519. http://onlinelibrary.wiley.com/cochranelibrary/

Odent, M. (1992). *The nature of birth and breastfeeding.* Westport, CT: Bergin and Garvey.

Poets, A., Steinfeldt, R., & Poets, C. F. (2011). Sudden deaths and severe apparent life-threatening events in term infants within 24 hours of birth. *Pediatrics, 127,* 869–873.

Prechtl, H. (1977). *The neurological examination of the full term new born infant. Clinics in developmental medicine, No. 63* (2nd ed.). London, United Kingdom: William Heinemann Books Ltd.

Righard, L., & Alade, M. O. (1990). Effect of delivery room routines on success of first breast-feed. *The Lancet, 336,* 1105–1107.

Righard, L., & Frantz, K. (1992). *Delivery self-attachment* [DVD]. Pasadena, CA: Geddes Productions, Available from http://www.geddesproduction.com

Riordan, J. (2010). Anatomy and physiology of lactation. In J. Riordan, & K. Wambach (Eds.), *Breastfeeding and human lactation (4th ed.).* Sudbury, MA: Jones & Bartlett Learning.

Skadberg, B. T., Morild, I., & Markestad, T. (1998). Abandoning prone sleeping: Effects on the risk of sudden infant death syndrome. *Journal of Pediatrics, 132,* 340–343.

Smillie, C. M., Frantz, K., & Makelin, I. (2007) *Baby-led breastfeeding* [DVD]. Pasadena, CA: Geddes Productions. Available from http://www.geddesproduction.com

Stark, D. (2011). *Babybabyohbaby* [DVD]. Oakland, CA: Stark Productions. Available from http://www.babybabyohbaby.com/

Thoresen, M., Cowan, F., & Whitelaw, A. (1988). Effect of tilting oxygenation in newborn infants. *Archives of Diseases of Childhood,* 63, 315–317.

Touwen, B. C. L. (1984). Primitive reflexes—conceptual or semantic problem? In F. R. Prechtl (Ed.), *Continuity of neural functions from prenatal to postnatal life* (pp. 115–125). London, United Kingdom: MacKeith Press.

UNICEF UK Baby Friendly Initiative. (2010). *Skin-to-skin contact.* Retrieved from http://www.unicef.org.uk/BabyFriendly / Resources/Training-resources/E-learning-for-GPs/

UNICEF/WHO Baby-Friendly USA. (2012). *Photo 1 in skin-to-skin contact.* Retrieved from http://www.unicef.org.uk/ BabyFriendly/ Parents/Resources/AudioVideo/

Uvnäs-Moberg, K. (1989). The gastrointestinal tract in growth and reproduction. *Scientific American, 7,* 60–65.

Watson Genna, C. (2013). *Supporting sucking skills* (2nd ed.). Burlington, MA: Jones & Bartlett Learning.

Widström, A. M. (1988). *Studies on breast-feeding: Behaviour and peptide hormone release in mothers and infants. Applications in delivery and maternity ward care* (Unpublished master's thesis). Karolinska Institute, Stockholm, Sweden.

Widström, A. M. (1996). *Breastfeeding: Baby's choice* [DVD]. Stockholm, Sweden: Liber Utbildning. Available from http://www.worldcat.org/title/breastfeeding-babys-choice/oclc/300431320

Widström, A. M. (2013). *Breast crawl: Initiation of breastfeeding by breast crawl a scientific overview.* Retrieved from http://www.breastcrawl.org/science.shtml

Widström, A. M., Lilja, G., Aaltomaa-Michalias, P., Dahllof, A., Lintula, M., & Nissen, E. (2011). Newborn behaviour to locate the breast when skin-to-skin: A possible method for enabling early self-regulation. *Acta Paediatrica Scandinavica, 100,* 79–85.

Widström, A. M., Ransjo-Arvidson, A. B., Christensson, K., Matthiesen, A. S., Winberg, J., & Uvnäs-Moberg, K. (1987). Gastric suction in healthy newborn infants: Effects on circulation and developing feeding behavior. *Acta Paediatrica Scandinavica, 76,* 566–572.

Widström, A. M., Wahlberg, V., Matthiesen, A. S., Eneroth, P., Uvnäs-Moberg, K., Werner, S., & Winberg, J. (1990). Shortterm effects of early suckling and touch of the nipple on maternal behaviour. *Early Human Development, 21,* 153–163.

Winberg, J. (1995). Viewpoint: Examining breastfeeding performance: Forgotten influencing factors. *Acta Paediatrica, 84,* 465–467.

YouTube. (2014). Retrieved from https://www.youtube.com/results?search_query=breast+crawl

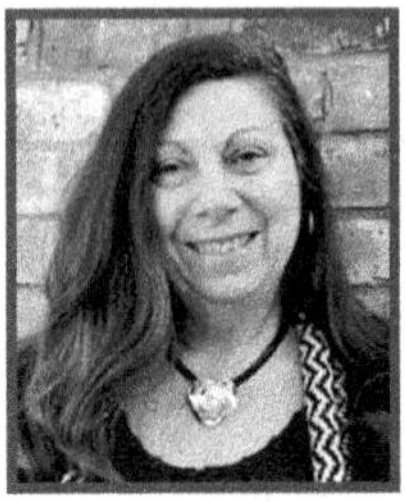

Suzanne Colson, PhD, MSc, BA, is a midwife and a nurse. Her thesis introduced a new paradigm called Biological Nurturing™ and won the prestigious English Royal College of Nursing Inaugural Akinsanya Award for originality and scholarship in doctoral studies. Suzanne is an Akinsanya scholar 2007, a former senior lecturer at Canterbury Christ Church University, and co-founder of The Nurturing Project—an organization created to disseminate Biological Nurturing research. She is an honorary member, and a founding mother/leader of La Leche League France. She is also on the professional advisory board of La Leche League of Great Britain. She has more than 35 years clinical experience supporting breastfeeding mothers, first in France, working with Dr. Michel Odent, then in London hospitals as a caseload midwife and midwife/lactation specialist, and finally during her research appointments and university work as a senior midwifery researcher and lecturer. Suzanne is the author of numerous articles, research papers, a book, and three DVDs. Retired from the university and active midwifery practice, she remains available for clinical consultation and lectures widely across the world.

Formula Supplementation of the Breastfed Infant Assault on the Gut Microbiome

Marsha Walker, RN, IBCLC, RLC[1]

Keywords: breastfeeding, infant formula hazards, infant gut microbiota, immunological programming

Although formula supplementation is well known to have detrimental effects on the duration and exclusivity of breastfeeding, on the maternal milk production, and on the health outcomes of mothers and infants, there are immediate and long-lasting effects on the infant's gut microbiome. Breast milk is an important element modulating the metabolic and immunological programming relative to a child's health. An unfavorable or abnormal microbial colonization during early life interferes with many functions in the gut and facilitates invasion of pathogens and foreign or harmful antigens. Alterations of the gut environment (such as from supplementation with formula) are directly responsible for mucosal inflammation and disease, autoimmunity conditions, and allergic disorders in childhood and adulthood. Clinicians and parents will benefit from knowledge of this side effect of formula supplementation.

1 Marshalact@gmail.com

Supplementation of breastfed infants has a history and tradition dating back to ancient times. Currently, the 2013 Breastfeeding Report Card from the Centers for Disease Control and Prevention shows that even though 76.5% of infants born in the U.S. have "ever" been breastfed, nearly a quarter of them receive formula supplementation before 2 days of age. In some states, up to 35% of newborns receive formula supplementation within 48 hours of birth. Mothers may supplement with formula because of perceived or real insufficient milk production, to settle a fussy baby, to assure that the baby is satisfied and getting enough, to obtain more sleep, at the suggestion of a health care provider for a medical or non-medical indication, because her friends or family members engage in this practice, or from pressure to do so.

Mothers may also fall prey to infant formula manufacturers' promotion of a formula specifically labeled for supplementing breastfed infants, and believe unfounded claims that the use of this product will result in longer breastfeeding durations. Receipt of formula discharge bags when mothers leave the hospital furthers the notion of formula supplementation as necessary, sanctioned by the health care system, and something that "everyone" does. Although it is well known that formula supplementation decreases the duration of breastfeeding (Bolton, Chow, Benton, & Olson, 2009), reduces maternal milk supply, and increases the risk for abandonment of breastfeeding (Hall et al., 2002), there is a side effect of which few mothers and clinicians are aware: the immediate alteration in the newborn gut microbiome.

The Infant Gut Microbiome

The microbiota in the human gut (intestine) is an immense and diverse community of microorganisms. The bulk of these microorganisms are bacteria whose vital role is in the development of intestinal functions that affect the lifelong health of an individual. Gut microbiota influence the growth and differentiation of the gut's epithelial cells (the cells that line the intestine), and are critical to nutritive, metabolic, immunological, and protective functions. The number of bacterial cells in the gastrointestinal tract greatly exceeds the number of human cells in the body. The total quantity of genes in the various bacterial species far outnumber the amount of human genes by more than 100-fold.

The totality of gut microorganisms, their genetic elements, and their environmental interactions is known as the microbiome. This gut microbiome has been called an "organ within an organ," or a "super organ," because it has and performs its own functions. These functions include executing enzymatic reactions and modulating gene expression involved in mucosal barrier fortification, forming new blood vessels, and promoting intestinal maturation following birth.

The central nervous system is also affected through gut-brain communication pathways, with alterations in gut microbiota implicated in certain brain disorders, such as autistic spectrum disorder (Heijtz et al., 2011; Kang et al., 2013). Thus, bacteria regulate the development of the intestinal barrier, as well as its functions, and are important, even in distant body organs. The gut is the largest interface between the body and the world outside it, containing 60% to 70% of the immune system. Its numerous roles facilitate absorption of nutrients while acting as a barrier to prevent pathogens, toxins, and antigens from entering the body and causing acute or chronic diseases and conditions. Illness and conditions associated with intestinal barrier dysfunction are more common in adults who were formula-fed as infants compared with those who were breastfed (Verhasselt, 2010).

The gut's physical barrier is the first line of defense, and is composed of a layer of columnar epithelial cells between which are the tight junctions. The tight junctions control gut permeability, allowing the passage of fluids, electrolytes, and small macromolecules, but preventing the passage of larger macromolecules. The gut is permeable during fetal life and early after birth. Gut closure, or closure of the tight junctions, starts during the first postnatal week. Any delay, change, or insult to the gut that changes this process predisposes the infant to infection, inflammatory states, and allergic sensitization (Maheshwari & Zemlin, 2009). The gut closure process is mediated by hormones and growth factors in human milk that facilitate epithelial growth and maturation.

Breastfed and formula-fed infants demonstrate a marked and impressive differences in their respective gut microbiota (Mountzouris, McCartney, & Gibson, 2002). Compared with formula-fed infants, breastfed infants develop a lower gut pH (acidic environment) of approximately 5.1–5.4 throughout the first 6 weeks of life, which is dominated by Bifidobacterium, and a reduced population of pathogenic (disease-causing) microbes, such as numerous species of *Escherichia coli,* Bacteroides, clostridia, enterococci, and streptococci. Supplementation with formula induces a rapid shift in the gut bacterial pattern of a breastfed infant. The dominance of bifidobacteria during exclusive breastfeeding decreases when infant formula is added to the diet (Favier, Vaughan, De Vos, & Akkermans, 2002). If breastfed infants receive infant formula supplementation during the first 7 days of life, the production of a strongly acidic gut environment is delayed, and its full potential may never be reached.

Breastfed infants who receive supplements develop gut flora and behavior such as those of formula-fed infants. The probability of an infant being appropriately colonized by bifidobacteria is reduced when the mother has a high body mass index, the mother experiences excessive weight gain during pregnancy, and the baby is delivered by cesarean section. The likelihood of appropriate bifidobacterial colonization is higher when the mother is of normal weight, has appropriate bifidobacterial colonization in her own gut and in her breast milk, and is actively breastfeeding (Isolauri, 2012). Breast milk is thought to be one of the most important postpartum elements modulating the metabolic and immunological programming relative to a child's health (Aaltonen et al., 2011).

Breast milk is not sterile, nor is it meant to be. Researchers have identified more than 700 bacterial species in human milk that vary from mother to mother depending on mode of delivery and the BMI of the mother. Colostrum has an even higher diversity of bacterial species than does transitional or mature milk (Cabrera-Rubio et al., 2012). Beneficial bacteria are directly transported to the baby's gut by breast milk, whereas the oligosaccharides in breast milk support the growth of these bacteria. Non-human oligosaccharides added to infant formula are structurally different from human oligosaccharides and do not appear to be functionally equivalent. Breast milk promotes bacterial growth in aggregate form, whereas formula promotes growth as single cells. Growth of single cells in the porous gut barrier of the newborn is potentially much more detrimental than is the growth of much larger aggregates (Zhang, Lee, Truneh, Everett, & Parker, 2012). The early bacterial colonizers regulate the gene expression of the cells lining the digestive tract because they create a favorable environment for themselves that function to inhibit the growth of other harmful bacteria.

Just One Bottle

It has been known for many years that relatively small amounts of formula given to breastfed infants (one supplement per 24 hours) result in shifts from a breastfed to a formula-fed gut flora pattern (Bullen, Tearle, & Stewart, 1977; Mackie, Sghir, & Gaskins, 1999). With the introduction of supplementary formula, the flora becomes almost indistinguishable from normal adult flora within 24 hours (Gerstley, Howell, & Nagel, 1932). If breast milk were again given exclusively, it would take 2 to 4 weeks for the intestinal environment to return to a state favoring the gram-positive flora (Brown & Bosworth, 1922; Gerstley et al., 1932).

It is thought that initial sensitization to food allergens in the exclusively breastfed infant may occur from external sources, such as a single feeding of infant formula. In susceptible families, breastfed infants can be sensitized to cow's milk protein by the giving of "just one bottle" (inadvertent supplementation, unnecessary supplementation, or planned supplementation) in the newborn nursery during the first 3 days of life (Cantani & Micera, 2005; Host, 1991; Host, Husby, & Osterballe, 1988). The feeding of a cow's milk-based infant formula as a supplement to breastfeeding in the hospital has been shown to increase the risk of cow's milk allergy, as does occasional exposure to cow's milk formula during the first 8 weeks following discharge (Saarinen et al., 2000). Infant formula supplementation may also be associated with the development of type 1 diabetes in susceptible infants. This may occur as a result of inflammation in the gut and/or the increased permeability of the gut when it encounters cow's milk-based infant formula (Knip, Virtanen, & Akerblom, 2010).

Perturbations to the normal healthy colonization patterns of the gut can result in lifelong disease (Di Mauro et al., 2013). Such perturbations can be specifically caused by the use of infant formula, which changes the gut's bacterial population. Breast milk's protective action relies mainly on its ability to modulate intestinal microflora composition during the early days of life (Guaraldi & Salvatori, 2012). The early bacterial colonizers of the infant's gut regulate the gene expression of the cells that line the digestive tract, creating a favorable environment for themselves, which inhibits the growth of potentially pathogenic bacteria. Even small amounts of formula supplementation of breastfed infants will result in shifts from a breastfed microbiota pattern to a formula-fed pattern (Mackie et al., 1999). The prudent clinician may wish to avoid giving breastfed babies formula in the hospital and before gut closure occurs, unless there is a specific medical reason to do so.

Clinical Implications

A reduced or abnormal colonization of the infant gut during the first months of life (which can result from supplements of infant formula) provokes a slower maturation of the epithelial cell barrier functions, alters gut permeability, and consequently facilitates the invasion of pathogens and foreign or harmful antigens (Perrier & Corthesy, 2011). Nutrition during this time frame has a profound effect on the shape and trajectory of the body's microbiome.

Preterm infants are at an even higher risk when breast milk is supplemented with infant formula. Preterm infants already experience a high risk for acquiring necrotizing enterocolitis because of their lower gastric acid production, reduced ability to break down toxins, and low levels of secretory immunoglobulin A (SIgA), which increase bacterial adherence to the intestinal mucosa.

Taylor, Basile, Ebeling, and Wagner (2009) studied 62 preterm infants and demonstrated that those infants receiving more than 75% of their diet as breast milk had significantly lower intestinal permeability compared with formula-fed infants or those who received only small amounts of breast milk. The dose of breast milk became even more important over time because more than 25% of the diet needed to be breast milk at 30 days of age to still see a significant advantage. Preterm infants cannot fully digest carbohydrates and proteins. Undigested casein, a protein in infant formula, can function as a chemoattractant for neutrophils, exacerbating the inflammatory response, and opening the tight junctions between intestinal epithelial cells; disrupting the integrity of the epithelium barrier; and allowing the delivery of whole bacteria, endotoxin, and viruses directly into the bloodstream (Claud & Walker, 2001).

Feeding preterm infants with infant formula may produce colonization of the intestine with pathogenic bacteria, resulting in an exaggerated inflammatory response. The SIgA from colostrum, transitional milk, and mature milk (which is absent in infant formula) coats the gut, preventing attachment and invasion of pathogens by competitively binding and neutralizing bacterial antigens. This passively provides immunity during a time of reduced neonatal gut immune function.

Helping Mothers Understand

Helping mothers understand this specific side effect of formula supplementation is important. Clinicians can take advantage of teachable opportunities, both prenatally and postpartum. Scripting conversations may be helpful, such as examples in Table 1.

Table 1. Sample Scripts Regarding Side Effects on the Gut Microbiome of Formula Supplementation

Teachable Opportunities	Sample Script
Prenatal Obstetric visits Breastfeeding/childbirth classes WIC visits Social media/electronic resources Mothers' groups Publications/blogs/handouts	• "It's important that your baby gets just breast milk. Most of the immune system lives in the gut. Breast milk directs how good bacteria are lured to the gut and bad bacteria are routed into the diaper." • "Formula supplements can mess up the programming of the immune system and increase the chances of bowel infections, allergies, obesity, diabetes, and other diseases and conditions." • "Formula is not the same as breast milk, and its ingredients do not act the same as what is in breast milk."
Postpartum Mother wants to do both. Mother thinks she does not have enough milk, baby is not satisfied after feedings, baby cries when put down, or mother wants baby to sleep.	• "Your milk has all the vitamins and ingredients that your baby needs. Adding formula if it is not needed can disrupt the development of baby's immune system." • "I am concerned that adding formula will upset the process of programming baby's immune system. Let me see if I can help with what is troubling you." • "With your family history of diabetes I am uneasy about giving the baby formula."

In the Hospital

Formula supplementation that is started in the hospital is often continued post-discharge. There are several interventions that hospitals can take to reduce the amount of supplementation that is not medically indicated:

- » Infant formula bottles can be stored in a special or locked cabinet where nurses must sign out each bottle, recording the name of the patient, why the bottle is being given, and the name of the nurse or clinician who obtains the bottle.
- » Some hospitals have put formula bottles in their medication distribution system, such as a Pyxis system. This demonstrates that formula supplementation is to be used in a manner similar to medication, that is, only when medically necessary. This system can track formula usage and serve to indicate where additional staff education may be necessary.
- » Staffing of International Board Certified Lactation Consultants should follow the recommendations of the United States Lactation Consultant Association (USLCA), with patient ratios of 1.3 lactation consultants (LCs) per 1,000 births in a Level I hospital, 1.6 LCs per 1,000 births in a Level II hospital, and 1.9 LCs per 1,000 births in a Level III hospital (USLCA, 2010).
- » Mothers' own expressed colostrum or expressed breast milk are the first choices, should supplemen-

tation become necessary. Pasteurized donor human milk would be the next choice in the hospital. If formula must be used, then a hydrolyzed formula rather than a standard cow's milk-based formula would be a better choice (Committee on Nutrition, American Academy of Pediatrics, 2000). This would hopefully reduce the risk of alterations of the gut microbiome.

» Hospital staff should be educated regarding the side effects of formula supplementation of breastfed infants. Staff are ethically and legally responsible for acting in the best interests of their patients.

» Discharge bags from formula companies should not be distributed to mothers upon leaving the hospital. These represent another form of pressure to supplement breastfeeding infants with a product that is potentially harmful.

» Infant formula samples pose a potential risk to the infant, staff, and institution because powdered formula is not sterile, instructions are seldom provided regarding how to safely reconstitute or use the product in the discharge bag, and the hospital has no mechanism to inform patients if there is a recall of the formula sample.

As health care professionals, we can provide direct and honest communication and guidelines to the mothers and infants entrusted to our care. We owe them no less.

References

Aaltonen, J., Ojala, T., Laitinen, K., Poussa, T., Ozanne, S., & Isolauri, E. (2011). Impact of maternal diet during pregnancy and breastfeeding on infant metabolic programming: A prospective randomized controlled study. *European Journal of Clinical Nutrition, 65,* 10–19.

Bolton, T. A., Chow, T., Benton, P. A., & Olson, B. H. (2009). Characteristics associated with longer breastfeeding duration: An analysis of a peer counseling support program. *Journal of Human Lactation, 25,* 18–27.

Brown, E. W., & Bosworth, A. W. (1922). Studies of infant feeding XVI. A bacteriological study of the feces and the food of normal babies receiving breast milk. *American Journal of Diseases of Children, 23,* 243–258.

Bullen, C. L., Tearle, P. V., & Stewart, M. G. (1977). The effect of humanized milks and supplemented breast feeding on the faecal flora of infants. *Journal of Medical Microbiology, 10,* 403–413.

Cabrera-Rubio, R., Collado, M. C., Laitinen, K., Salminen, S., Isolauri, E., & Mira, A. (2012). The human milk microbiome changes over lactation and is shaped by maternal weight and mode of delivery. *American Journal of Clinical Nutrition, 96,* 544–551.

Cantani, A., & Micera, M. (2005). Neonatal cow milk sensitization in 143 case-reports: Role of early exposure to cow's milk formula. *European Review for Medical and Pharmacological Sciences, 9,* 227–230.

Centers for Disease Control and Prevention. (2013). *Breastfeeding report card: United States/2013.* Retrieved from http://www.cdc.gov/breastfeeding/pdf/2013BreastfeedingReportCard.pdf

Claud, E. C., & Walker, W. A. (2001). Hypothesis: Inappropriate colonization of the premature intestine can cause neonatal necrotizing enterocolitis. *FASEB Journal, 15,* 1398–1403.

Committee on Nutrition, American Academy of Pediatrics. (2000). Hypoallergenic infant formulas. *Pediatrics, 106,* 346–349.

Di Mauro, A., Neu, J., Riezzo, G., Raimondi, F., Martinelli, D., Francavilla, R., & Indrio, F. (2013). Gastrointestinal function development and microbiota. *Italian Journal of Pediatrics, 39,* 15. http://www.ijponline.net/content/39/1/15

Favier, C. F., Vaughan, E. E., De Vos, W. M., & Akkermans, A. D. L. (2002). Molecular monitoring of succession of bacterial communities in human neonates. *Applied and Environmental Microbiology, 68*, 219–226.

Gerstley, J. R., Howell, K. M., & Nagel, B. R. (1932). Some factors influencing the fecal flora of infants. *American Journal of Diseases of Children, 43*, 555–565.

Guaraldi, F., & Salvatori, G. (2012). Effect of breast and formula feeding on gut microbiota shaping in newborns. *Frontiers in Cellular and Infection Microbiology, 2*, 94.

Hall, R. T., Mercer, A. M., Teasley, S. L., McPherson, D. M., Simon, S. D., Santos, S. R., . . . Hipsh, N. E. (2002). A breast-feeding assessment score to evaluate the risk for cessation of breastfeeding by 7 to 10 days of age. *Journal of Pediatrics, 141*, 659–664.

Heijtz, R. D., Wang, S., Anuar, F., Qian, Y., Bjorkholm, B., Samuelsson, A., . . . Pettersson, S. (2011). Normal gut microbiota modulates brain development and behavior. *Proceedings of the National Academy of Science of the United States of America, 108*, 3047–3052.

Host, A. (1991). Importance of the first meal on the development of cow's milk allergy and intolerance. *Allergy Proceedings, 10*, 227–232.

Host, A., Husby, S., & Osterballe, O. (1988). A prospective study of cow's milk allergy in exclusively breastfed infants. *Acta Paediatrica Scandinavia, 77*, 663–670.

Isolauri, E. (2012). Development of healthy gut microbiota early in life. *Journal of Paediatrics and Child Health, 48* (3), 1–6.

Kang, D. W., Park, J. G., Ilhan, Z. E., Wallstrom, G., LaBaer, J., Adams, J. B., & Krajmalnik-Brown, R. (2013). Reduced incidence of Prevotella and other fermenters in intestinal microflora of autistic children. *PLoS One, 8*, e68322.

Knip, M., Virtanen, S. K., & Akerblom H. K. (2010). Infant feeding and the risk of type 1 diabetes. *American Journal of Clinical Nutrition, 91*, 1506S–1513S.

Mackie, R. I., Sghir, A., & Gaskins, H. R. (1999). Developmental microbial ecology of the neonatal gastrointestinal tract. *American Journal of Clinical Nutrition, 69*, 1035S–1045S.

Maheshwari, A., & Zemlin, M. (2009). Ontogeny of the intestinal immune system. *Haematologica Reports, 2* (10), 18–26.

Mountzouris, K. C., McCartney, A. L., & Gibson, G. R. (2002). Intestinal microflora of human infants and current trends for its nutritional modulation. *British Journal of Nutrition, 87*, 405–420.

Perrier, C., & Corthesy, B. (2011). Gut permeability and food allergies. *Clinical & Experimental Allergy, 41*, 20–28.

Saarinen, K. M., Juntunen-Backman, K., Järvenpää, A. L., Klemetti, P., Kuitunen, P., Lope, L., . . . Savilahti, E. (2000). Breast-feeding and the development of cows' milk protein allergy. *Advances in Experimental Medicine and Biology, 478*, 121–130.

Taylor, S. N., Basile, L. A., Ebeling, M., & Wagner, C. L. (2009). Intestinal permeability in preterm infants by feeding type: Mother's milk versus formula. *Breastfeeding Medicine, 4*, 11–15.

United States Lactation Consultant Association. (2010). *International board certified lactation consultant staffing recommendations for the inpatient setting.* Retrieved from http:// uslca.org/wp-content/uploads/2013/02/IBCLC_Staffing_Recommendations_July_2010.pdf

Verhasselt, V. (2010). Neonatal tolerance under breastfeeding influence. *Current Opinion in Immunology, 22* (5), 623–630.

Zhang, A. Q., Lee, S. Y. R., Truneh, M., Everett, M. L., & Parker, W. (2012). Human whey promotes sessile bacterial growth, whereas alternative sources of infant nutrition promote planktonic growth. *Current Nutrition and Food Science, 8*, 168–176.

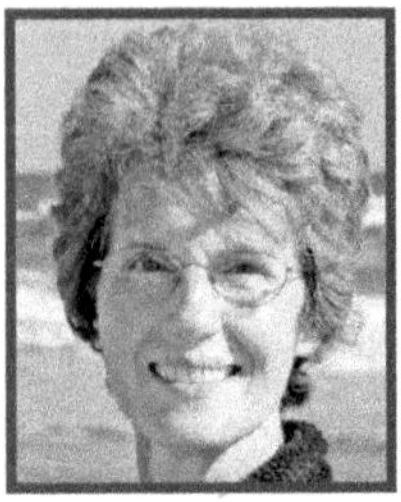

Marsha Walker, RN, IBCLC, RLC, is a registered nurse and an International Board Certified Lactation Consultant. She has been assisting breastfeeding families in hospital, clinic, and home settings since 1976. Marsha is the executive director of the National Alliance for Breastfeeding Advocacy: Research, Education, and Legal Branch. She is a board member of the Massachusetts Breastfeeding Coalition, the United States Lactation Consultant Association (USCLA), and BabyFriendly USA; and USLCA's representative to the U.S. Department of Agriculture's Breastfeeding Promotion Consortium. Marsha is the author of numerous publications, including *Breastfeeding Management for the Clinician: Using the Evidence.*

Decreased Breastfeeding as One Factor on a Short List That Causes Pandemics of Allergic and Autoimmune Disease

William Parker, PhD[1]
Emily Foltz
Angela Q. Zhang

Keywords: breastfeeding, human biome, autoimmunity, allergy

Postindustrial society is plagued with pandemics of noninfectious, immune-related illnesses. These diseases, which include allergic, autoimmune, and neuroinflammatory diseases, are not found in preindustrial societies, and are apparently caused by a limited number of environmental factors. These factors, essentially incompatible with human genetics, are each associated with a wide range of immune diseases. The most influential of these factors is a loss of diversity from the ecosystem of the human body, a condition termed "biome depletion." This state affects all postindustrial humans during and after fetal development, and remains the strongest challenge for modern medicine to overcome in the field of immunology. Fortunately, progress is being made. On the

1 bparker@duke.edu, Department of Surgery, Duke University Medical Center, Durham, NC

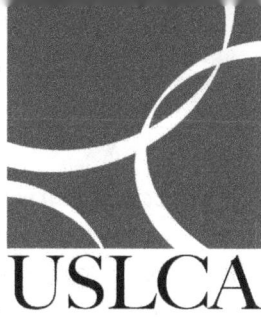

other hand, other factors associated with pandemics of allergic and autoimmune disease are within the control of each individual rather than the medical establishment. These factors include unrequited or chronic psychological stress, vitamin D deficiency, and substitution of breast milk with infant formula. Decreased breastfeeding in particular has a profound effect on immunity, probably through multiple mechanisms that involve increased stress levels, alterations of the human biome, and direct modulation of the immune system by mechanisms that remain largely uncharacterized. Given the synergism of these factors that adversely affect immunity in postindustrial culture, the importance of avoiding as many of these factors as possible is emphasized.

Pandemics of Noninfectious, Immune-Related Diseases Limited to Postindustrial Culture

Postindustrial society faces an onslaught of diseases related to overreactive immune systems. This immune reactivity toward harmless foreign (extrinsic) or self (intrinsic) targets leads to allergic and autoimmune diseases, respectively. Consequently, up to 40% of the U.S. population suffers from allergic disorders (Arbes, Gergen, Elliott, & Zeldin, 2005; A. H. Liu et al., 2010), and another 3% suffers from autoimmune conditions (Jacobson, Gange, Rose, & Graham, 1997). Furthermore, several maladies that affect cognitive function—including migraine headaches, schizophrenia, and autism—may be induced by aberrant immune responses (Becker, 2007; Bilbo, Jones, & Parker, 2012; Fan, Goff, & Henderson, 2007; Parker, Perkins, Harker, & Muehlenbien, 2012; Patterson, 2009; Waeber & Moskowitz, 2005). Of critical importance is the observation that pandemics of this family of noninfectious, immune-related diseases do not occur in preindustrial societies (Bickler & DeMaio, 2008). Not only were the diseases not described in antiquity, but they also remain absent in preindustrial cultures of today (Bickler & DeMaio, 2008).

Given these observations, it can readily be concluded that these pandemics are not caused by genetics but are rather caused by changes in the postindustrial environment that are incompatible with human health. In other words, the rapid changes introduced by postindustrial culture are essentially incompatible with our genetics, which remain relatively unchanged since the beginning of the industrial revolution. This mismatch between our genes and our environment is widely appreciated as the cause of postindustrial pandemics of obesity, heart disease, and type 2 diabetes.

Just as high-calorie diets without exercise lead to obesity-associated diseases, so does a handful of factors in our environment lead to noninfectious, immune-related diseases. These environmental factors are associated with both allergic and autoimmune disease, indicating that factors that lead to one type of disease also lead to the other. For example, substituting infant formula for breast milk not only increases the risk of many allergies, including eczema (Chandra, Puri, & Hamed, 1989; Merrett et al., 1988), it also increases the incidence of autoimmune diseases, such as multiple sclerosis (Ryder et al., 1991) and type 1 diabetes (Fava, Leslie,

& Pozzilli, 1994). Although substituting infant formulas for breast milk is an important factor leading to immune disease, this factor is joined by a handful of other factors that also drive postindustrial immune systems toward the same hyperreactive, pathogenic state.

Triggers for Disease and Associated Genetics Are Not the Cause of the Pandemics

Before describing postindustrial factors that cause pandemics of allergic and autoimmune disease, it is first important to point out that these diseases have two important contributors that are independent, or at least partially independent, of the postindustrial environment. The first of these two is called the "trigger." Triggers include a wide range of very common substances. For example, ragweed pollen serves as a trigger for hay fever, and viral infections can serve as a trigger for several immunemediated conditions, including autism and multiple sclerosis. However, since ragweed pollen and viruses have been around for millennia without causing these diseases, and since these triggers are largely unavoidable, triggers are not generally a cause of postindustrial pandemics, and it is not the avoidance of triggers that is important for the prevention and, in many cases, the treatment of disease.

On the other hand, toxins and pollutants can also trigger immune disease (Rea, 1988), and these are associated with industrialization. However, it is the postindustrial society, typically less polluted than societies in the peak of their industrialization, which has the most immune disease. Thus, it is expected that toxins and pollutants are not the actual cause of disease, although they can serve as triggers. The fact that inflammation associated with immune disorders can impair toxin metabolism (Bilbo et al., 2012) further exacerbates the roles of toxins in immune disease, but based on the epidemiology of disease, it is probably not these toxins that cause the pandemic of disease.

Independent of triggers, genetics has also been identified as a contributor to pandemics of postindustrial, immune-related diseases. Almost all allergic and autoimmune diseases are linked to one or more genetic factors present in the population. However, genetics, like many triggers, is essentially independent of the postindustrial environment, and thus cannot be the causative factor for any postindustrial pandemic. Thus, in a very real sense, the search for genetic links to postindustrial immune disease is of little practical use. Not only is genetics not the cause of the pandemic, but effective treatment of many mutation-induced diseases (e.g., cystic fibrosis, sickle cell anemia, Tay-Sachs disease, and color blindness) has proven extremely difficult for modern medicine.

Cultural Factors Leading to Pandemics of Noninfectious, Immune-Related Diseases

Looking beyond long-established triggers and genetics, assessment of the scientific and medical literature points toward a very limited number of factors that appear to be the cause of recently emerging diseases. These factors involve changes in our culture so that human genetics no longer match the human environment. These changes have profoundly affected the "ecosystem of the human body," and all of the organisms associated with that ecosystem, called "the human biome."

At present, four cultural factors have been identified that alter the human biome, making it susceptible to allergic and autoimmune disease. Data from anthropologic, immunologic, epidemiologic, and clinical studies support these cultural factors as underlying causes of allergic and autoimmune disease (Bilbo, Wray, Perkins, & Parker, 2011; Parker et al., 2012). In all cases except one, causal links have been unequivocally demonstrated by clinical studies. These four are as follows:

1. ***The alteration or complete loss of living species normally associated with the human biome*** is the primary factor leading to pandemics of allergic and autoimmune disease. The use of modern toilets, water-treatment facilities, and modern medicine is largely responsible for this factor called "biome depletion." For example, the use of toilets

has eliminated most symbiotic helminths (worms) from the human body. Although generally thought of as parasites, some of these helminths are, in fact, harmless when found in postindustrial culture, and modulate the immune system effectively, preventing immune-related disease. A vast body of scientific evidence, including data from clinical studies, studies in animal models, and studies in basic-science laboratories, strongly supports this view in a manner that is overwhelming. This information has been reviewed in detail recently (Bilbo et al., 2011; Parker et al., 2012), and will be summarized only briefly here.

The introduction of sewage systems, water-treatment facilities, and modern medicine into postindustrial society all but eliminated many infectious diseases and parasites. Unfortunately, this vitally important advance in public health has produced an unexpected and profoundly negative backlash: the human immune system, which has leaned into an onslaught of infectious parasites for all of human existence, is now destabilized by the sudden removal of its old adversaries.

In ecological terms, the species we lost from our body's ecosystem turned out to be "keystone": without them, the system destabilizes. Fortunately, this realization suggests that "biome reconstitution," the controlled reintroduction of appropriate organisms, could effectively combat immune disease. Unfortunately, there is very little to be done about this problem now by the average person. Not only would abandonment of hygienic practices in postindustrial culture lead to widespread infectious disease, but also the needed organisms are already gone. Worse hygiene will not establish helminths that are entirely absent in the population, and even if it could, no one envisions curing allergic and autoimmune disease by restoring widespread infectious disease. Thus, short of obtaining organisms outside the bounds of traditional medical practice (a practice increasing in popularity), or participating in experimental clinical trials, a cure for immune disease involving biome reconstitution must wait on modern medicine to re-introduce the missing organisms in a controlled and safe fashion.

Fortunately, this factor is only one of four factors, and the other three factors listed in the following text (Figure 1) can be controlled by the typical individual. Because this first factor is out of our immediate control, it is extremely important to control the other three. The immune system already has one big strike against it, so further strikes should be avoided if at all possible.

2. ***Unrequited or chronic psychological stress*** is well established as a factor that increases the incidence

of both allergic and autoimmune disease in postindustrial cultures (Bagnasco, Bossert, & Pesce, 2006; Bailey et al., 2009; Buret, 2006; Glaser & Kiecolt-Glaser, 2005; Gouin, Hantsoo, & KiecoltGlaser, 2011; Ippoliti et al., 2006; Kiecolt-Glaser et al., 2009; Moylan et al., 2013; Reiche, Nunes, & Morimoto, 2004; Stojanovich & Marisavljevich, 2008). Using experimental models, the causal link between chronic psychological stress and immune dysfunction, as well as some of the underlying biochemical/immunological pathways involved, have been established (Bailey et al., 2009).

Figure 1. Postindustrial Factors Undermining Immune Function

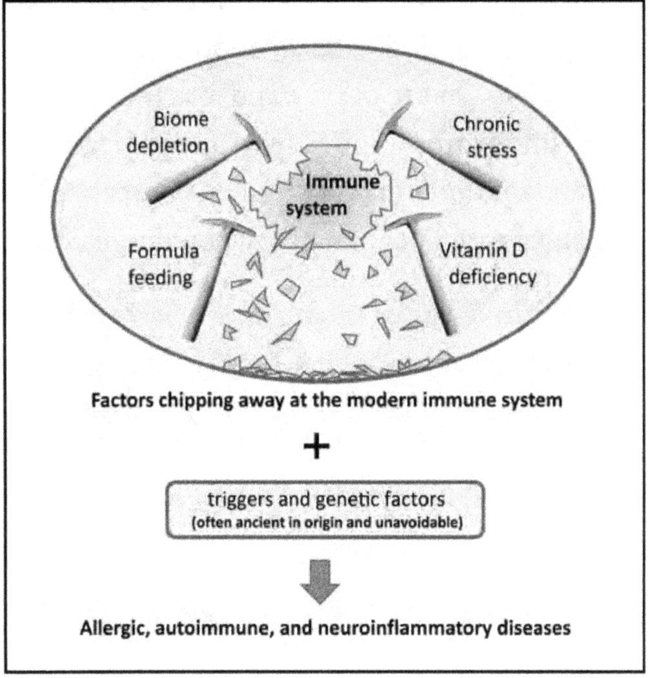

However, it is unclear whether Western culture is particularly prone to psychological compared to preindustrial (agrarian and hunter-gatherer) cultures, but it is clear that increased psychological stress is bad for our immune health. Thus, various stress-reduction strategies are recommended for restoring immune health and combating allergic and autoimmune disease.

Various factors associated with postindustrial culture undermine immune function and increase the chances of a wide range of inflammatory diseases, including allergic and autoimmune diseases. Biome depletion, as described in the text, is probably the single most important factor undermining immune function, and modern medicine is still grappling with an approach to resolve this problem. On the other hand, other factors known to undermine immune function are largely avoidable and include the lack of breastfeeding in a substantial portion of the population.

3. ***Vitamin D deficiency,*** like the other factors described earlier, causes an increase in the incidence of both allergic and autoimmune conditions (Cannell, 2008; de Borst et al., 2011; N. Q. Liu et al., 2011; Lucas et al., 2011; Mark & Carson, 2006; Sharief, Jariwala, Kumar, Muntner, & Melamed, 2011; Wagner, Taylor, & Hollis, 2008). Hossein-Nezhad, Spira, and Holick (2013) have solidly established the link between immune dysfunction

and vitamin D deficiency, probing a wide range of immune factors impaired by vitamin D deficiency and demonstrating that normalization of vitamin D levels can reverse disease. As stated recently by Holick (HosseinNezhad et al., 2013):

Our data suggest that any improvement in vitamin D status will significantly affect expression of genes that have a wide variety of biologic functions of more than 160 pathways linked to cancer, autoimmune disorders, and cardiovascular disease that have been associated with vitamin D deficiency. This study reveals for the first time molecular finger prints that help explain the non-skeletal health benefits of vitamin D.

Inadequate levels of vitamin D were probably relatively rare before the industrial revolution, when sunlight was the main source of light for almost all human activity. In contrast, the use of windows that block ultraviolet (UV) light, sunscreen, and indoor lighting devoid of UV light has left more than half of the postindustrial population lacking in adequate vitamin D (Holick, 2006). Although sporadic exposure to the sun, which causes severe sunburn and subsequent skin cancer, is not a recommended means of avoiding this problem, vitamin D supplements are readily available and quite effective (Hollis, Johnson, Hulsey, Ebeling, & Wagner, 2011). At present, the primary hurdle in overcoming this factor is educational in nature. Even many health care professionals are unaware that vitamin D deficiency puts individuals at risk for anything more than bone density problems, despite the preponderance of evidence (Staud, 2005; Wagner et al., 2008) supporting the view that vitamin D deficiency increases the risk for immune-related disease.

4. ***Replacement of mother's milk with infant formula,*** as mentioned earlier, is yet another factor that apparently affects both allergic and autoimmune disease. Indeed, the potential ramifications of replacing breast milk with infant formula for human biology are vastly complex. However, unlike the first three factors described earlier, the effect of substituting formula for breast milk cannot readily be subjected to controlled clinical trials, and has not been investigated using experimental-animal models. Nevertheless, the role of breastfeeding in immunity is supported by a wide range of evidence, and from several perspectives, that evidence points toward a lack of breast milk as a contributing factor in the pandemics of immune disease.

The Impact of Human Milk on Immune Function

Clinical studies demonstrate conclusively that human milk is vitally important for immune function. At the same time, immunological and biological studies lag behind, and our understanding of the role of breast milk in human biology is in its infancy. Nevertheless, current research suggests that the impact of human milk on immune function is multifactoral. One key point of impact appears to be the importance of human milk in establishing the bacteria within a baby's gastrointestinal tract. It is upon these bacteria that the development of the immune system is critically dependent (Gaskins, Croix, Nakamura, & Nava, 2008; Tsuji, Suzuki, Kinoshita, & Fagarasan, 2008).

Human milk and infant formulas lead to a much different microbial population in the infant digestive tract (for a review, see Guaraldi & Salvatori, 2012). In general, the bacteria in the gut of babies fed infant formula more closely resemble the bacteria found in adults rather than those found in normal (breastfed) infants (Mackie, Sghir, & Gaskins, 1999). Thus, babies fed infant formula rather than breast milk are essentially bypassing steps in the development of their bacterial symbionts, called the microbiome. This alteration of the microbiome may be important for immune function because the development of the microbiome is very closely tied to the development of immunity. For example, animals that are raised with no microbiome have an immune system that is grossly underdeveloped (for a review, see Tlaskalová-Hogenová et al., 2002).

Simple in vitro experiments readily show the profound differences between human milk and infant formulas in terms of their interactions with bacteria (Zhang, Lee, Truneh, Everett, & Parker, 2012). Human milk facilitates the clumping of bacteria, reducing the numbers of free-floating bacteria, whereas infant formulas have the opposite effect: they induce the rapid proliferation of free-swimming bacteria. The results of a typical experiment are shown in Figure 2.

Both nutritional sources induce bacteria to grow, but they cause the bacteria to grow in profoundly different ways. The copious quantities of secretory IgA (SIgA) in human milk, but not infant formulas, are probably responsible, at least in part, for this observation (Bollinger et al., 2003).

Figure 2. Effect of Infant Nutrition on Friendly Bacteria

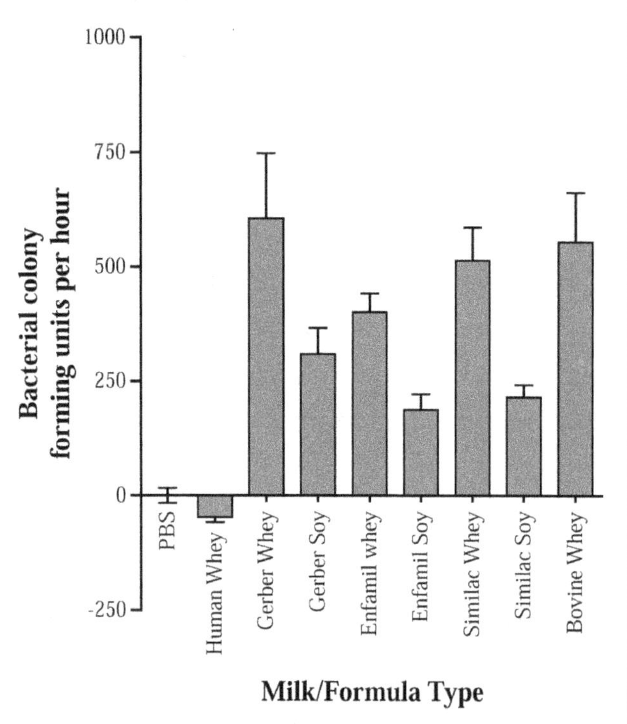

Evidence suggesting that SIgA supports the growth of living films of bacteria, called biofilms, in the normal, healthy gut was first uncovered about a decade ago (Bollinger et al., 2003). For example, artificial models of the human gut containing both human gut cells and bacterial biofilms were first successfully created using a nutrient broth containing SIgA (Bollinger et al., 2006). Previous attempts at creating the artificial system without SIgA were unsuccessful.

Human milk proteins have a profoundly different effect on the growth of growth of non-pathogenic E. coli compared to other forms of infant nutrition. The increase in colony forming units per hour was measured following a 2-hr incubation at physiologic temperature (37 °C). Phosphate buffered saline (PBS) was used as a "control" (the number of bacteria present after incubation with a nutrient-deficient liquid), and the number of colony forming units under those conditions were set at zero. Whereas human milk proteins (Human Whey) caused an actual decrease in the number of bacterial counts, other forms of infant nutrition caused a dramatic increase. These experiments and a larger series of related experiments have been described previously (Zhang et al., 2012), and demonstrate that not only does human milk support the growth of E. coli, but that it supports it in a fashion much differently than does other forms of infant nutrition. Importantly, the decrease in colony counts because of human milk proteins was caused by clumping of growing bacteria, not by killing of bacteria.

A second means by which breast milk alters immune function is probably through the modulation of psychological stress. As pointed out earlier, chronic psychological stress is one of a very limited number of factors that leads to allergic and autoimmune disease (Figure 1). Breastfeeding not only reduces psychological stress in the infant, but is also associated with reduced stress in the mother (Groër, 2005; Hahn-Holbrook, Holt-Lunstad, Holbrook, Coyne, & Lawson, 2011; Mezzacappa, 2004). In this case, the act of breastfeeding may be as important as the breast milk itself. The idea has recently, but strongly and convincingly, emerged that skin-to-skin contact between mother and newborn, a usual component of breastfeeding, is by itself extremely important for both infant and maternal psychological well-being (Acolet, Sleath, & Whitelaw, 1989; Gray, Watt, & Blass, 2000; Ludington-Hoe et al., 1999; LudingtonHoe, Hashemi, Argote, Medellin, & Rey, 1992).

In one dramatic example, Morgan and colleagues found that the simple act of separating mothers from their newborns for only one-hour apparently induces a substantial increase in psychological stress in the newborn (Morgan, Horn, & Bergman, 2011). In that study, the authors evaluated healthy infants with and without a 1-hr separation from their mother, providing convincing evidence suggesting that separation from the mother is not compatible with human biology. The authors conclude that such separation "may not be benign."

To what extent skin-to-skin contact with the mother versus the actual breast milk affects maternal and infant well-being remains largely unknown and presents an extremely important area for future investigation. However, it is evident that, especially in the infant, breastfeeding reduces psychological stress, one of the leading factors associated with allergic and autoimmune disease.

Conclusions

By the time a human baby is born in postindustrial society, he or she has already been exposed to an environment (the womb) affected by biome depletion. In addition, there is a substantial possibility that the same infant has already been exposed to the effects of chronic psychological stress and vitamin D deficiency in the womb. To be deprived of breast milk at this point adds further to the potential milieu of insults already suffered by the infant's immune system, and seems worth avoiding if at all possible.

Breastfeeding involves a vastly complex connection with mother and infant, affecting the entire body, including the immune, endocrine, nervous, and digestive systems. Perhaps just as importantly, breastfeeding affects establishment of the human biome, particularly the microbiome, which is intimately tied to the immune system development. Given that breastfeeding has been the established method of providing infant nutrition for as long as humanity has existed, it seems unsurprising that alteration of this process leads to an increased incidence of disease.

Although the biochemical and physiologic reasons that breastfed babies have a reduced risk for noninfectious immune-related disease remain largely unknown, studies are beginning to emerge that explain, at least in part, this connection. Perhaps one of the most important considerations regarding the modern decrease in breastfeeding should be that other factors associated with postindustrial society operate synergistically with deprivation from mother's milk to induce immune-related disease. Fortunately, some of those factors can be avoided using vitamin D supplements as needed and by reducing chronic stress as much as possible.

On the other hand, biome depletion, caused by necessary developments in sanitation and medical practice, remains uncontrolled at present, and work toward reversing this problem is in its infancy. The ubiquitous nature of biome depletion in postindustrial society and the potent damage this factor has on immune function argues strongly in favor of avoiding, if at all possible, factors such as deprivation from mother's milk, which further damage immune function.

References

Acolet, D., Sleath, K., & Whitelaw, A. (1989). Oxygenation, heart rate and temperature in very low birthweight infants during skin-to-skin contact with their mothers. *Acta Paediatrica Scandinavica, 78,* 189–193.

Arbes, S. J., Jr., Gergen, P. J., Elliott, L., & Zeldin, D. C. (2005). Prevalences of positive skin test responses to 10 common allergens in the US population: Results from the Third National

Health and Nutrition Examination Survey. *Journal of Allergy Clinical Immunology, 116*, 377–383.

Bagnasco, M., Bossert, I., & Pesce, G. (2006). Stress and autoimmune thyroid diseases. *Neuroimmunomodulation, 13*, 309–317.

Bailey, M. T., Kierstein, S., Sharma S., Spaits, M., Kinsey, S. G., Tliba, O., & Haczku, A. (2009). Social stress enhances allergen-induced airway inflammation in mice and inhibits corticosteroid responsiveness of cytokine production. *The Journal of Immunology, 183*, 3551.

Becker, K. G. (2007). Autism, asthma, inflammation, and the hygiene hypothesis. *Medical Hypotheses, 69*, 731–740.

Bickler, S. W., & DeMaio, A. (2008). Western diseases: current concepts and implications for pediatric surgery research and practice. *Pediatric Surgery International, 24*, 251–255.

Bilbo, S. D., Jones, J. P., & Parker, W. (2012). Is autism a member of a family of diseases resulting from genetic/cultural mismatches? Implications for treatment and prevention. *Autism Research and Treatment, 2012*, 1–11.

Bilbo, S. D., Wray, G. A., Perkins, S. E., & Parker, W. (2011). Reconstitution of the human biome as the most reasonable solution for epidemics of allergic and autoimmune diseases. *Medical Hypotheses, 77*, 494–504.

Bollinger, R. R., Everett, M. L., Palestrant, D., Love, S. D., Lin, S. S., & Parker W. (2003). Human secretory immunoglobulin A may contribute to biofilm formation in the gut. *Immunology, 109*, 580–587.

Bollinger, R. R., Everett, M. L., Wahl, S. D., Lee, Y. H., Orndorff, P. E., & Parker W. (2006). Secretory IgA and mucin-mediated biofilm formation by environmental strains of Escherichia coli: Role of type 1 pili. *Moleculor Immunology, 43*, 378–387.

Buret, A. G. (2006). How stress induces intestinal hypersensitivity. *American Journal of Pathology, 168*, 3–5.

Cannell, J. J. (2008). Autism and vitamin D. *Medical Hypotheses, 70*, 750–759.

Chandra, R. K., Puri, S., & Hamed, A. (1989). Influence of maternal diet during lactation and use of formula feeds on development of atopic eczema in high risk infants. *BMJ, 299*, 228–230.

de Borst, M. H., de Boer, R. A., Stolk, R. P., Slaets, J. P. J., Wolffenbuttel, B. H. R., & Navis G. (2011). Vitamin D deficiency:

Universal risk factor for multifactorial diseases? *Current Drug Targets, 12*, 97–106.

Fan, X., Goff, D. C., & Henderson, D. C. (2007). Inflammation and schizophrenia. *Expert Review of Neurotherapeutics, 7*, 789–796.

Fava, D., Leslie R. D., & Pozzilli P. (1994). Relationship between dairy product consumption and incidence of IDDM in childhood in Italy. *Diabetes Care, 17*, 1488–1490.

Gaskins, H. R., Croix, J. A., Nakamura, N., & Nava, G. M. (2008). Impact of the intestinal microbiota on the development of mucosal defense. *Clinical Infectious Disease, 46*, S80–S86.

Glaser, R., & Kiecolt-Glaser, J. K. (2005). Stress damages immune ssytem and health. *Discovery Medicine, 5*, 165–169.

Gouin, J. P., Hantsoo, L. V., & Kiecolt-Glaser, J. K. (2011). Stress, negative emotions, and inflammation. In J. T. C. J. Decety (Ed.), *Handbook of social neurosciences* (pp. 814–829). New York, NY: Wiley.

Gray, L., Watt, L., & Blass, E. M. (2000). Skin-to-skin contact is analgesic in healthy newborns. *Pediatrics, 105*, e14.

Groër, M. W. (2005). Differences between exclusive breastfeeders, formula-feeders, and controls: A study of stress, mood, and endocrine variables. *Biological Research for Nursing, 7*, 106–117.

Guaraldi, F., & Salvatori, G. (2012). Effect of breast and formula feeding on gut microbiota shaping in newborns. *Frontiers in Cellular and Infection Microbiology, 2*, 94. http://dx.doi. org/10.3389/fcimb.2012.00094

Hahn-Holbrook, J., Holt-Lunstad, J., Holbrook, C., Coyne, S. M., & Lawson, E. T. (2011). Maternal defense: Breastfeeding increases aggression by reducing stress. *Psychological Science, 22*, 1288–1295.

Holick, M. F. (2006). Resurrection of vitamin D deficiency and rickets. *Journal of Clinical Investigation*, 116, 2062–2072.

Hollis, B. W., Johnson, D., Hulsey, T. C., Ebeling, M., & Wagner, C. L. (2011). Vitamin D supplementation during pregnancy: Double-blind, randomized clinical trial of safety and effectiveness. *Journal of Bone & Mineral Research, 26*, 2341–2357.

Hossein-Nezhad, A., Spira, A., & Holick, M. F. (2013). Influence of Vitamin D Status and Vitamin D: Supplementation on genome wide expression of white blood cells: A randomized doubleblind clinical trial. *PLoS One, 8*, e58725.

Ippoliti, F., De Santis, W., Volterrani, A., Canitano, N., Frattolillo, D., Lucarelli, S., . . . Frediani, T. (2006). Psychological stress affects response to sublingual immunotherapy in asthmatic children allergic to house dust mite. *Pediatric Allergy and Immunology, 17,* 337–345.

Jacobson, D. L., Gange, S. J., Rose, N. R., & Graham, N. M. (1997). Epidemiology and estimated population burden of selected autoimmune diseases in the United States. *Clinical Immunology and Immunopathology, 84,* 223–243.

Kiecolt-Glaser, J. K., Heffner, K. L., Glaser, R., Malarkey, W. B., Porter, K., Atkinson, C., . . . Marshall, G. D. (2009). How stress and anxiety can alter immediate and late phase skin test responses in allergic rhinitis. *Psychoneuroendocrinology, 34,* 670–680.

Liu, A. H., Jaramillo, R., Sicherer, S. H., Wood, R. A., Bock, S. A., Burks, A. W., . . . Zeldin, D. C. (2010). National prevalence and risk factors for food allergy and relationship to asthma: Results from the National Health and Nutrition Examination Survey 2005-2006. *Journal of Allergy and Clinical Immunology, 126,* 798–806.e13.

Liu, N. Q., Kaplan, A. T., Lagishetty, V., Ouyang, Y. B., Ouyang, Y., Simmons, C. F., . . . Hewison, M. (2011). Vitamin D and the regulation of placental inflammation. *Journal of Immunology, 186,* 5968–5974.

Lucas, R. M., Ponsonby, A. L., Dear, K., Valery, P. C., Pender, M. P., Taylor, B. V., . . . McMichael, A. J. (2011). Sun exposure and vitamin D are independent risk factors for CNS demyelination. *Neurology, 76,* 540–548.

Ludington-Hoe, S. M., Anderson, G. C., Simpson, S., Hollingsead, A., Argote, L. A., & Rey, H. (1999). Birth-related fatigue in 34-36week preterm neonates: Rapid recovery with very early kangaroo (skin-to-skin) care. *Journal of Obstetric, Gynecologic, and Neonatal Nursing, 28,* 94–103.

Ludington-Hoe, S. M., Hashemi, M. S., Argote, L. A., Medellin, G., & Rey, H. (1992). Selected physiologic measures and behavior during paternal skin contact with Colombian preterm infants. *Journal of Developmental Physiology, 18,* 223–232.

Mackie, R. I., Sghir, A., & Gaskins, H. R. (1999). Developmental microbial ecology of the neonatal gastrointestinal tract. *American Journal Clinical Nutrition, 69,* 1035S–1045S.

Mark, B. L., & Carson J. A. (2006). Vitamin D and autoimmune disease: Implications for practice from the multiple sclerosis literature. *Journal of the American Dietetic Association, 106,* 418–424.

Merrett, T. G., Burr, M. L., Butland, B. K., Merrett, J., Miskelly, F. G., & Vaughan-Williams, E. (1988). Infant feeding and allergy: 12-month prospective study of 500 babies born into allergic families. *Annals of Allergy, 61,* 13–20.

Mezzacappa, E. S. (2004). Breastfeeding and maternal stress response and health. *Nutrition Reviews, 62,* 261–268.

Morgan, B. E., Horn, A. R., & Bergman, N. J. (2011). Should neonates sleep alone? *Biological Psychiatry, 70,* 817–825.

Moylan, S., Eyre, H. A., Maes, M., Baune, B. T., Jacka, F., & Berk, M. (2013). Exercising the worry away: How inflammation, oxidative and nitrogen stress mediates the beneficial effect of physical activity on anxiety disorder symptoms and behaviours. *Neuroscience & Biobehavioral Review, 13,* 37(4), 573–584.

Parker, W., Perkins, S. E., Harker, M., & Muehlenbein, M. P. (2012). A prescription for clinical immunology: The pills are available and ready for testing. *Current Medical Research and Opinion, 28,* 1193–1202.

Patterson, P. H. (2009). Immune involvement in schizophrenia and autism: Etiology, pathology and animal models. *Behavior & Brain Research, 204,* 313–321.

Rea, W. J. W. (1988). Chemical hypersensitivity and the allergic response. *Ear Nose Throat Journal, 67,* 50–56.

Reiche, E. M., Nunes, S. O., & Morimoto, H. K. (2004). Stress, depression, the immune system, and cancer. *Lancet Oncology, 5,* 617–625.

Ryder, R. W., Manzila, T., Baende, E., Kabagabo, U., Behets, F., Batter, V., . . . Heyward, W. L. (1991). Evidence from Zaire that breast-feeding by HIV-1-seropositive mothers is not a major route for perinatal HIV-1 transmission but does decrease morbidity. *AIDS, 5,* 709–714.

Sharief, S., Jariwala, S., Kumar, J., Muntner, P., & Melamed, M. L. (2011). Vitamin D levels and food and environmental allergies in the United States: Results from the National Health and Nutrition Examination Survey 2005-2006. *Journal of Allergy & Clinical Immunology, 127,* 1195–1202.

Staud, R. (2005). Vitamin D: More than just affecting calcium and bone. *Current Rheumatology Reports, 7,* 356–364.

Stojanovich, L., & Marisavljevich, D. (2008). Stress as a trigger of autoimmune disease. *Autoimmunity Review, 7,* 209–213.

Tlaskalová-Hogenová, H., Tucková, L., Lodinová-Zádniková, R., Stepánková, R., Cukrowska, B., Funda, D. P., . . . Sánchez, D. (2002). Mucosal immunity: Its role in defense and allergy. *International Archives of Allergy & Immunology, 128,* 77–89.

Tsuji, M., Suzuki, K., Kinoshita, K., & Fagarasan, S. (2008). Dynamic interactions between bacteria and immune cells leading to intestinal IgA synthesis. *Seminars in Immunology, 20,* 59–66.

Waeber, C., & Moskowitz, M. A. (2005). Migraine as an inflammatory disorder. *Neurology, 64,* S9–S15.

Wagner, C. L., Taylor, S. N., & Hollis, B. W. (2008). Does vitamin D make the world go 'round'? *Breastfeeding Medicine, 3,* 239–250.

Zhang, A. Q., Lee, S. Y. R., Truneh, M., Everett, M. L., & Parker, W. (2012). Human whey promotes sessile bacterial growth, whereas alternative sources of infant nutrition promote planktonic growth. *Current Nutrition & Food Science, 8,* 168–176.

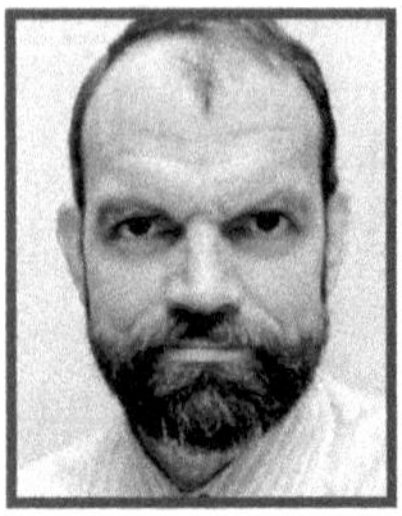

William Parker, PhD, is an Associate Professor in the Department of Surgery at Duke University Medical Center. He is best known for the discovery of the function of the human appendix and for work on immunity in wild animals. His most recent work combines medical research with fundamental biology, ecology, anthropology, and immunology, providing potential solutions for pandemics of allergic and autoimmune diseases.

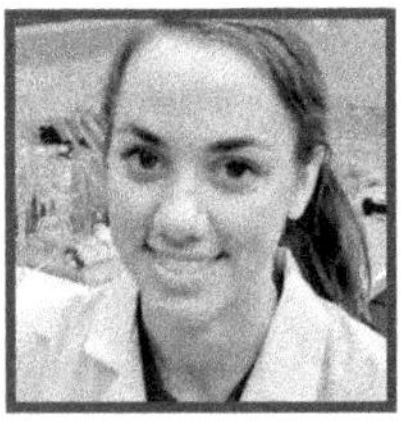

Emily Foltz is a senior at Duke University, majoring in Biology. Her current research involves comparing the effects of various pasteurization methods on the functional properties of breast milk, particularly regarding its interaction with gut bacteria.

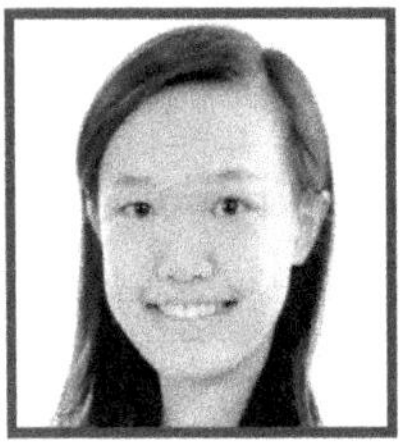

Angela Zhang is a junior at the Massachusetts Institute of Technology, majoring in Biology. Her published work was the first to demonstrate profound differences between infant formulas and breast milk in terms of their ability to support microbial biofilms.

USLCA

Breastfeeding Management for the Late Preterm Infant

Practical Interventions for "Little Imposters"

Marsha Walker, RN, IBCLC, RLC[1]

Keywords: late preterm, breastfeeding difficulties, jaundice, dehydration

Infants who are late preterm (34–36 weeks) may appear mature, but they are physiologically, metabolically, and neurologically immature. Late preterm infants are at higher risk for a number of problems, including poor feeding, jaundice, hospital re-admittance, and potential breastfeeding failure. This article provides specific strategies for working with late preterm infants and avoiding these negative health outcomes.

Introduction

Sara was born at 35 weeks, weighing 6 pounds, 6 ounces. Her mother Anna was told that Sara was considered "full term" because of her weight, and was even sent home early because she was so "big and healthy." Sara had a

1 Executive Director, National Alliance for Breastfeeding Advocacy

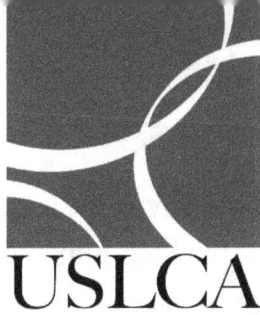

good latch, but tired quickly at the breast. Three days later, Sara was readmitted for high bilirubin levels and weight loss. Anna's milk supply was blamed, and she was advised to start formula.

This unfortunate scenario is played out all too often, but does not have to be the outcome for the breastfed late-preterm infant.

The rate of premature births (<37 weeks) in the United States is 12.3% (Martin et al., 2010), with the largest portion of these being the late preterm infant (34–36 weeks). The 8.8% rate of late preterm births places over 450,000 infants at risk for respiratory distress, apnea, bradycardia, excessive sleepiness, weight loss, dehydration, feeding difficulties, weak sucking, jaundice, hypoglycemia, hypothermia, immature self-regulation, sepsis, hospital readmission (Adamkin, 2006; Engle et al., 2007), prolonged formula supplementation, and breastfeeding failure.

Every Week is Important

Even though some late preterm infants may look like full-term infants and weigh between 4.5 and > 7 pounds, they are physiologically, metabolically, and neurologically immature, which is why they are often referred to as "little imposters." While all of the organ systems have formed, the brain and respiratory system are among the last to mature. During the last 6 weeks of gestation, subcutaneous tissue and brown fat are laid down, glycogen stores increase in the liver, antibodies are passed to the fetus, and fetal muscle tone increases. Interruption in these processes helps explain the late preterm infant's susceptibility to hypothermia, hypoglycemia, and sepsis. Low muscle tone affects the infant's ability to generate a vacuum at the breast (Kent et al., 2008).

An infant born at 34–35 weeks has 60% of the brain mass of a term infant. At 36 weeks, the brain weight is about 80% of the size of a full-term infant (Kinney, 2006). The immature brain stem negatively impacts upper airway and lung volume control, laryngeal reflexes, and the chemical control of breathing and sleep mechanisms. Interruption in brain development and myelinization helps explain the late preterm infants' sleepiness, difficulty with state control, and uncoordinated sucking and breathing.

Human Milk as a Brain Builder

Human milk is extremely important to late preterm infants, as it provides a rich source of components specially designed for brain growth:

» Increased brain ganglioside and glycoprotein sialic acid concentration in human milk-fed infants enhances developmental outcomes compared with formula-fed infants (Wang et al., 2003). Human milk oligosaccharides are an important source of sialic acid. Formula-fed infants receive only 20% of the sialic acid that a breastfed infant receives and are unable to synthesize the difference.

» Lactose (galactose+glucose) in breastmilk ensures an abundant supply of galactocerebrosides that are needed for myelinization of the brain. Infants fed soy formula or lactose-free cow's milk formula consume a diet lacking particular brain growth nutrients.

» Late preterm infants, just like early preterm infants (<34 weeks), are vulnerable to conditions associated with oxidative stress, such as necrotizing enterocolitis, and respiratory distress syndrome. Breastmilk has a much higher antioxidative capacity than infant formula and helps neutralize oxidative stress in young babies (Ezaki et al., 2008).

Meeting the Feeding Challenges of the Late Preterm Infant

Late preterm infants present a number of feeding challenges, including fewer and shorter awake periods, sleepiness, tiring easily when feeding, have a weak suck and low tone, and may have an inability to sustain sucking, fatiguing easily before finishing a feeding. They are easily overstimulated and may shut down before consuming adequate amounts of milk. They may take small volumes of milk during the early days in the hospital, which may be sufficient for that period of time, but are unable to consume higher volumes of milk, post-discharge. Their tone may be adequate at the start of a feeding, but rapidly decreases during the feeding, indicating decreased endurance. They may go through the motions of feeding, moving their jaw up and down, but low tone generally translates to poor vacuum, often resulting in little, if any, milk transfer.

Breastfeeding Interventions for the Inpatient Stay

The First Hour

If the infant and mother are clinically stable, the infant should be placed skin-to-skin on the mother's chest and assisted to breastfeed within the first hour of birth.

Rationale: Late preterm infants show better cardiorespiratory stability with early skin-to-skin contact (Moore et al., 2007). A dose-response relationship exists between early skin-to-skin contact and exclusive breastfeeding, with longer contact times resulting in an increased likelihood of breastfeeding exclusivity in the hospital (Bramson et al., 2010). Early skin-to-skin contact reduces the risk of hypothermia and lowers the risk of hypoglycemia by decreasing crying (Christensson et al., 1992), and increasing breastfeeding opportunities.

The First Day

The infant should be put to breast frequently:

- Within an hour of birth
- Once every hour for the next 3 to 4 hours
- Every 2–3 hours until 12 hours of age

» At least 8 times or more each 24 hours during the hospital stay

Rationale: This feeding plan is designed for preventing hypoglycemia or for infants in the hypoglycemic range (California Diabetes and Pregnancy Program, 2002).

Positioning

Infants should be positioned in a cross cradle, clutch, or ventral (prone) position to breastfeed, avoiding the cradle hold.

Rationale: Late preterm infants are prone to positional apnea due to airway obstruction, increasing the risk of apnea, bradycardia, and oxygen desaturation in positions that create excessive flexion in the neck and trunk. They lack postural control in their necks and may have difficulty maintaining stability during feedings. Semi-reclined maternal positioning with the infant placed prone may improve ventilation and stimulate feeding reflexes (Colson et al., 2008).

Breastfeeding interventions should aim to accomplish three goals:

- Prevent adverse outcomes,
- Establish the mother's milk supply, and
- Assure adequate milk intake (Walker, 2008).

Breastfeeding care plans need to be created for the inpatient period, for discharge, and for any problems encountered or changes required once home (Walker, 2009).

Problems/Interventions

Use of the Dancer hand position helps stabilize the jaw to keep the infant from slipping off the nipple or from biting or clenching the jaw (Danner & Cerutti, 1984). For infants who do not demonstrate spontaneous mouth opening, or who do not open wide enough, the mother can gently exert downward pressure on the chin with her index finger as the infant approaches the breast (Figure 1).

Smacking sounds at the breast indicate loss of contact between the tongue and the nipple/areola. Sublingual pressure can be applied by the mother as she slips her index finger directly behind and under the tip of the chin where the tongue attaches, limiting the downward movement of the jaw.

Areolar edema may compromise latch. Use reverse pressure softening (Cotterman, 2004) or areolar compression (Miller & Riordan, 2004) to displace fluid away from the nipple and expose the nipple for an easier latch.

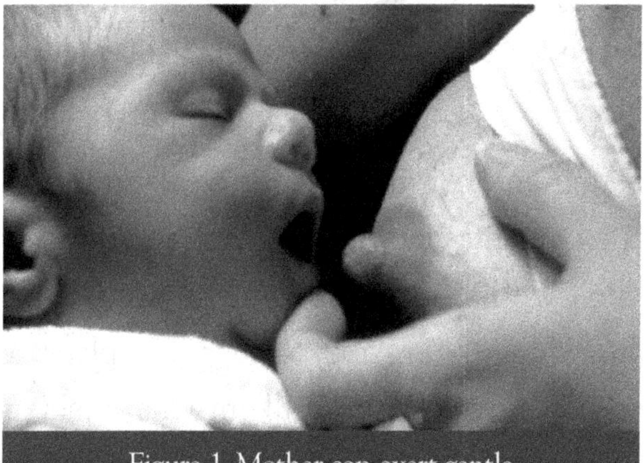

Figure 1. Mother can exert gentle downward pressure on the chin.

Flat nipples can be everted with a modified syringe (Kesaree et al., 1993) or commercial device designed to evert flat nipples.

Latch Incentives

For infants unable to latch independently, latch may be assisted with a milk-filled dropper or other tool, such as a syringe or tube feeding device. These may require another person's assistance. Placed at the side of the mouth as a latch is initiated, small boluses of colostrum or milk can be provided to initiate fluid flow, as flow regulates suck. Some infants engage in rapid side-to-side head movements, making latch difficult, painful, or impossible. As the infant is guided to the breast, touching the midline of the upper lip with the dropper will eliminate these movements and orient the baby to the breast (Figure 2). As the baby latches, placing a few drops of milk in the corner of the mouth will encourage a swallow followed by a nutritive suck (Figure 3).

If other latch techniques fail, a nipple shield may help initiate latch and compensate for weak sucking, as late preterm infants may lack the strength to draw the nipple/areola into their mouth and/or generate the -60mmHg of vacuum (Geddes et al., 2008) to keep it in place. Mothers can hand express colostrum/milk into the shield tunnel or pre-fill the tunnel using a periodontal or oral syringe for an immediate sucking reward.

Unsustained Sucking/Fatigue/Ineffective Milk Transfer

Alternate massage/breast compressions are helpful in sustaining sucking, compensating for weak vacuum, and increasing milk transfer. The breast is massaged and compressed during pauses between sucking bursts, which improves the pressure gradient between the breast and infant's mouth. Alternate massage is done on each side at each feeding until the infant no longer needs the extra assistance, taking care that the baby does not lose the latch. Care must be taken to assure that the volume compressed does not overwhelm the infant. For infants unable to transfer sufficient amounts of milk with alternate massage or with a nipple shield in place, a tube feeding device can be used or the tube from a tube feeding device can be run on top of or under the nipple shield to deliver pumped milk supplements.

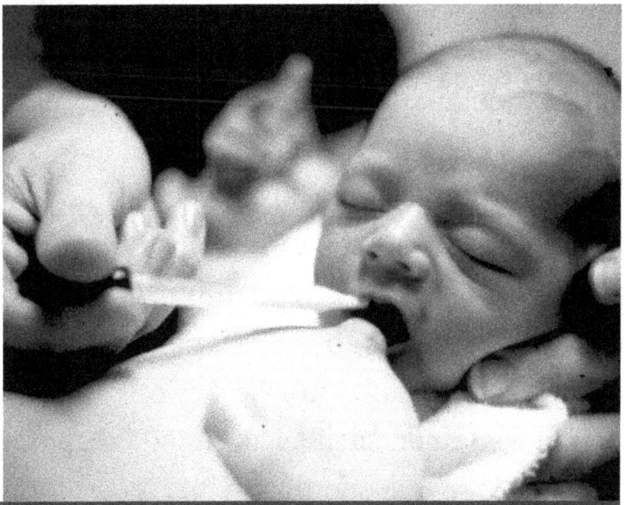

Figure 2. Dropper-assisted latch

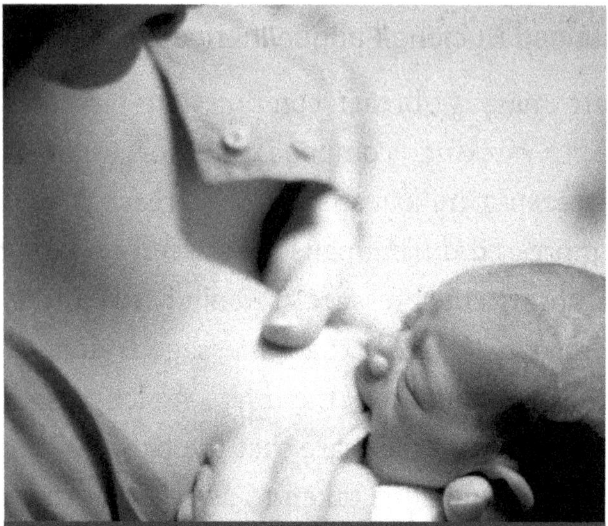

Figure 3. Milk incentive using a dropper

Supplementation

If the infant cannot obtain adequate colostrum/milk directly from the breast, with the use of frequent cue-based feeds, with the use of alternate massage, with milk incentives at the breast, or with a nipple shield in place, then supplementation may be necessary. Expressed colostrum/milk in volumes of 5-10 ml every 2 to 3 hours on day one, 10-20 ml on day 2, and 20-30 ml on day 3 are suggested as appropriate physiologic amounts (Stellwagen et al., 2007). Mothers can hand express colostrum into a teaspoon (5 ml) and spoon-feed this to the infant (Hoover, 1998). If mothers use a breast pump to collect colostrum, pumping into a small container, such as an Ameda diaphragm or Medela colostrum collection container, placed between the valve and collection bottle may yield a greater quantity of retrievable colostrum. Diabetic mothers may wish to bring prenatally expressed colostrum to the hospital should their infant need to be supplemented (Cox, 2006).

Milk Production: Initiation and Maintenance if the Infant is Unable to Feed Effectively at Breast or Mother and Baby are Separated

If the infant cannot gain appropriate weight by frequent feedings at the breast, or with the use of pumped hind-milk, or with fortified breastmilk, then infant formula may temporarily be needed. Use of a hydrolyzed formula reduces the risk of sensitizing susceptible infants to allergies (Greer et al., 2008) or diabetes and may also lower bilirubin levels (Gourley et al., 2005).

Supplementation may be provided by tube feeding devices at the breast, cups, finger feeding, droppers, syringes, or bottles. Cup feeding allows the participation of the masseter and temporalis muscles, similar to their functioning while feeding at the breast (Gomes et al., 2006). Use of artificial nipples may weaken sucking in an infant who already demonstrates diminished vacuum generation at the breast (Ferrante et al., 2006; Mizuno & Ueda, 2006). Finger feeding with a tube-feeding device requires the infant to generate a vacuum to remove milk, as biting actions will not release milk as they do with an artificial nipple.

Manual expression during the first 48 hours may yield more colostrum than with the use of an electric pump (Ohyama et al., 2010). Combined techniques of manual expression, breast compression, and use of an electric breast pump have been shown to improve milk yield in preterm mothers (Morton et al., 2009).

Other Resources

Evidence-based hospital breastfeeding protocols for late preterm infants.

» **California Perinatal Quality Care Collaborative.** Care and Management of the Late Preterm Infant Toolkit: Nutrition

» **The Academy of Breastfeeding Medicine.** Protocol #10: Breastfeeding the near–term infant (35 to 37 weeks gestation)

» **UC San Diego Health System Late Preterm Infant Protocol and patient resources**

References

Adamkin, D.H. (2006). Feeding problems in the late preterm infant. *Clinical Perinatology, 33,* 831–837.

Bramson, L., Lee, J.W., Moore, E., et al. (2010). Effect of early skin–to–skin mother–infant contact during the first 3 hours following birth on exclusive breastfeeding during the maternity hospital stay. *Journal of Human Lactation, 26,* 130–137.

California Diabetes and Pregnancy Program. (2002). *Sweet success: Guidelines for care.* http://www.cdph.ca.gov/programs/cdapp/Pages/default.aspx

Christensson, K., Siles, C., Moreno, L., et al. (1992). Temperature, metabolic adaptation and crying in healthy full–term newborns cared for skin–to–skin or in a cot. *Acta Paediatrica, 81,* 488–493.

Colson, S.D., Meek, J.H., & Hawdon, J.M. (2008). Optimal positions for the release of primitive neonatal reflexes stimulating breastfeeding. *Early Human Development, 84*, 441–449.

Cotterman, K.J. (2004). Reverse pressure softening: a simple tool to prepare areola for easier latching during engorgement. *Journal of Human Lactation, 20*, 227–237.

Cox, S.G. (2006). Expressing and storing colostrum antenatally for use in the newborn period. *Breastfeeding Review, 14*, 11–16.

Danner, S.C., & Cerutti, E.R. (1984). *Nursing your neurologically impaired baby.* Rochester, NY: Childbirth Graphics.

Engle, W.A., Tomashek, K.M., Wallman, C., & the Committee on Fetus and Newborn, American Academy of Pediatrics. (2007). Late preterm infants: A population at risk. *Pediatrics, 120*, 1390– 1401.

Ezaki, S., Ito, T., Suzuki, K., & Tamura, M. (2008). Association between total antioxidant capacity in breast milk and postnatal age in days in premature infants. *Journal of Clinical Biochemistry & Nutrition, 42*, 133–137.

Ferrante, A., Silvestri, R., & Montinaro, C. (2006). The importance of choosing the right feeding aids to maintain breastfeeding after interruption. *International Journal of Orofacial Myology, 32*, 58–67.

Geddes, D.T., Kent, J.C., Mitoulas, R., & Hartmann, P.E. (2008). Tongue movement and intra-oral vacuum in breastfeeding infants. *Early Human Development, 84*, 471–477.

Gomes, C.F., Trezza, E.M.C., Murade, E.C.M., & Padovani, C.R. (2006). Surface electromyography of facial muscles during natural and artificial feeding of infants. *Journal of Pediatrics (Rio J), 82*, 103–109.

Gourley, G.R., Li, Z., Kreamer, B.L., & Kosorok, M.R. (2005). A controlled, randomized, double-blind trial of prophylaxis against jaundice among breastfed newborns. *Pediatrics, 116*, 385–391.

Greer, F.R., Sicherer, S.H. Burks, A.W., American Academy of Pediatrics Committee on Nutrition, & American Academy of Pediatrics Section on Allergy and Immunology. (2008). Effects of early nutritional interventions on the development of atopic disease in infants and children: The role of maternal dietary restriction, breastfeeding, timing of introduction of complementary foods, and hydrolyzed formulas. *Pediatrics, 121,* 183–191.

Hoover, K. (1998). Supplementation of the newborn by spoon in the first 24 hours. *Journal of Human Lactation, 14,* 245.

Kent, J.C., Mitoulas, L.R., Cregan, M.D., et al. (2008). Importance of vacuum for breastmilk expression. *Breastfeeding Medicine, 3,* 11–19.

Kesaree, N., Banapurmath, C.R., Banapurmath, S., & Shamanur, K. (1993). Treatment of inverted nipples using a disposable syringe. *Journal of Humam Lactation, 9,* 27–29.

Kinney, H.C. (2006). The near–term (late preterm) human brain and the risk for periventricular leukomalacia: A review. *Seminars in Perinatology, 30,* 81–88.

Martin, J.A., Osterman, M.J.K., & Sutton, P.D. (2010). *Are preterm births on the decline in the United States? Recent data from the National Vital Statistics System. NCHS data brief, no 39.* Hyattsville, MD: National Center for Health Statistics.

Miller, V., & Riordan, J. (2004). Treating postpartum breast edema with areolar compression. *Journal of Human Lactation, 20,* 223– 226.

Mizuno, K., & Ueda, A. (2006). Changes in sucking performance from nonnutritive sucking to nutritive sucking during breast and bottle–feeding. *Pediatric Research, 59,* 728–731.

Moore, E.R., Anderson, G.C., & Bergman, N. (2007). Early skin–to–skin contact for mothers and their healthy newborn infants. *Cochrane Database of Systematic Reviews,* Jul 18, (3):CD003519.

Morton, J., Hall, J.Y., Wong, R.J., Thairu, L., Benitz, W.E., & Rhine, W.D. (2009). Combining hand techniques with electric pumping increases milk production in mothers of preterm infants. *Journal of Perinatology, 29,* 757–764.

Ohyama, M., Watabe, H., & Hayasaka, Y. (2010). Manual expression and electric breast pumping in the first 48 h after delivery. *Pediatrics International, 52,* 39–43.

Stellwagen, L.M., Hubbard, E.T., & Wolf, A. (2007). The late preterm infant: A little baby with big needs. *Contemporary Pediatrics,* November 1. http://goo.gl/NpdKmm

Walker, M. (2008). Breastfeeding the late preterm infant. *JOGNN, 37*, 692–701.

Walker, M. (2009). *Breastfeeding the late preterm infant: Improving care and outcomes.* Amarillo, TX: Hale Publishing.

Wang, B., McVeagh, P., Petocz, P., & Brand–Miller, J. (2003). Brain ganglioside and glycoprotein sialic acid in breastfed compared with formula–fed infants. *American Journal of Clinical Nutrition, 78*, 1024–1029.

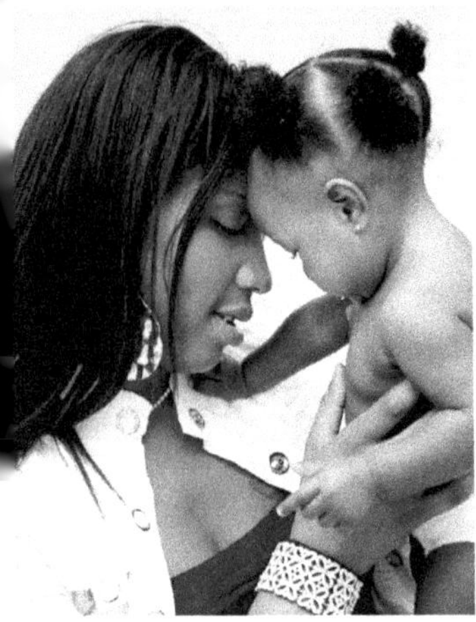

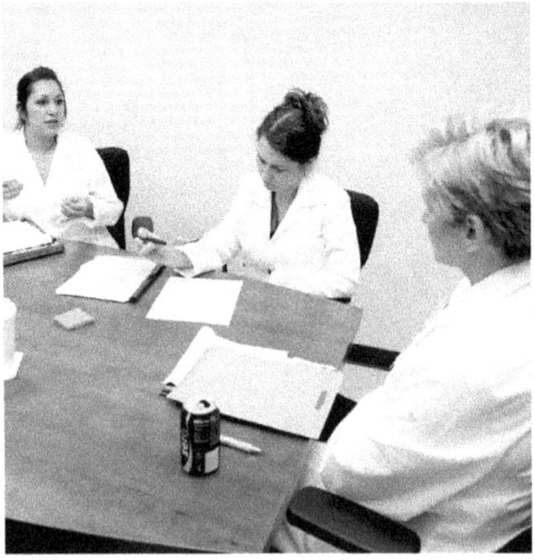

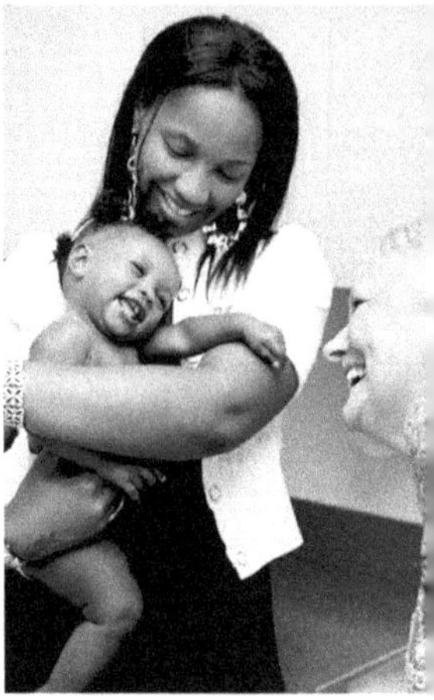

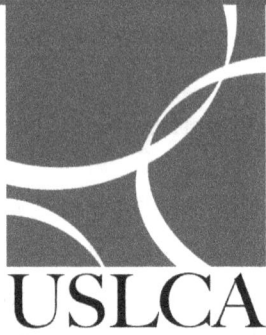

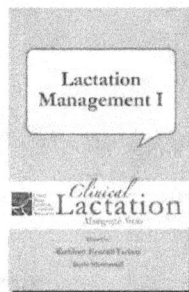

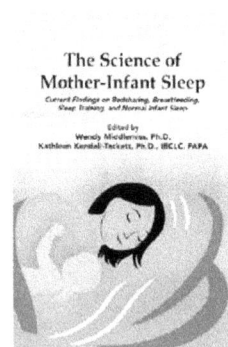

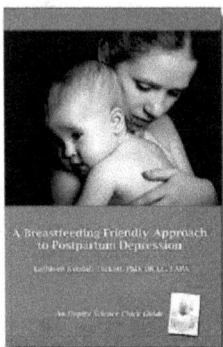

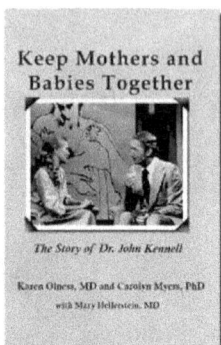

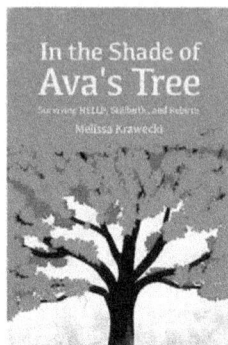

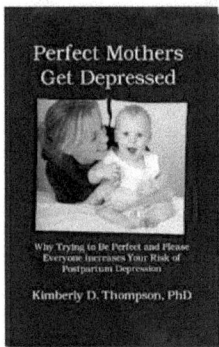

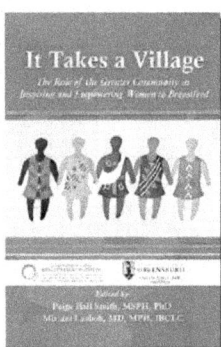

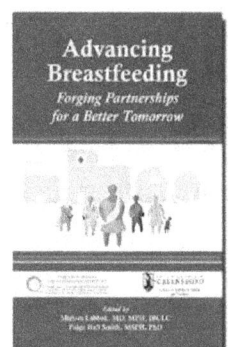

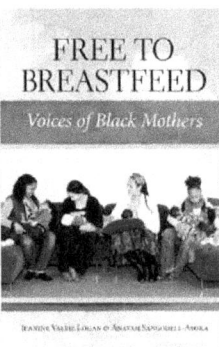

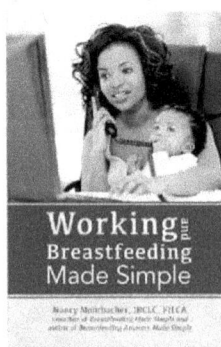

www.ingramcontent.com/pod-product-compliance
Lightning Source LLC
Chambersburg PA
CBHW060901280326
41934CB00007B/1134
* 9 7 8 1 9 3 9 8 0 7 3 6 6 *